MAJOR PROBLEMS IN INTERNAL MEDICINE

In Preparation

MAJOR PROBLEMS IN INTERNAL MEDICINE

Published

THOMAS R. CUPPS, M.D.

Clinical Associate
Laboratory of Immunoregulation
National Institute of Allergy and Infectious Diseases
National Institutes of Health
Bethesda, Maryland

ANTHONY S. FAUCI, M.D.

Chief, Laboratory of Immunoregulation
Deputy Clinical Director
National Institute of Allergy and Infectious Diseases
National Institutes of Health
Bethesda, Maryland

THE VASCULITIDES

VOLUME

XXI

IN THE SERIES

MAJOR PROBLEMS IN INTERNAL MEDICINE

Lloyd H. Smith, Jr., M.D., *Editor*

W. B. SAUNDERS COMPANY • PHILADELPHIA • LONDON • TORONTO • SYDNEY 1981

W. B. Saunders Company: West Washington Square
                            Philadelphia, PA   19105

                            1 St. Anne's Road
                            Eastbourne, East Sussex BN21 3UN, England

                            1 Goldthorne Avenue
                            Toronto, Ontario M8Z 5T9, Canada

                            9 Waltham Street
                            Artarmon, N.S.W. 2064, Australia

Library of Congress Cataloging in Publication Data

                                                    2/4/81
Cupps, Thomas R.

The vasculitides.

(Major problems in internal medicine; v. 21)

1. Vasculitis.   I. Fauci, Anthony S.   II. Title.
    Series. [DNLM: 1. Vasculitides.   2. Arteritis. W1
    MA492T v. 21 / WG 500 C974v]

RC694.5.I53C86   616.1'3   81–828

ISBN 0–7216–2794–3   AACR2

The Vasculitides   ISBN   0-7216-2794-3

Last digit is the print number: 9   8   7   6   5   4   3   2   1

To the patients of the Intramural Program of the National Institute of Allergy and Infectious Diseases, National Institutes of Health, who continue to teach us, and to Sheldon M. Wolff, M.D. for his encouragement and support during the formative stages of these studies.

FOREWORD

The human body has developed defense in depth against intruders whether animate or inanimate. Without this defense microorganisms would overwhelm us, in pursuit of what must seem like a maddeningly attractive package of nutrients. Defense is also directed against the foreignness of inanimate molecules when they are of sufficient size or special conformation to imply danger. In fact, it is their ability to trip the defense mechanism that defines them as antigens. Understanding of this silent armament is still incomplete. Even that which is known, however, reveals an impressive system to deliver defense to the appropriate locale, with appropriate force, for an appropriate period of time. There must be continuing and graduated retaliation rather than simply the release of a corporeal equivalent of nuclear warfare against every provocation.

In simpler days we had only "laudable pus"; later, inflammation could be conveniently summed up as rubor, tumor, and dolor. Now dolor best describes the predicament of the physician who attempts to understand the intricacies of host defense. Consider only briefly some of the weapon systems that are deployed. Immunocytes have a common cellular ancestry but then undergo very different higher education under thymus or bursa docents before taking up their respective commissions. They still engage in considerable sibling chatter, giving advice that can be loosely defined as helper or suppressor. This conversation by lymphokines is still obscure; no Rosetta stone is yet available. Antibodies are targeted on their respective antigens with remarkable specificity all spelled out in three-dimensional structures derived from variable region amino acids. But actually this weaponry turns out to have multiple warheads—the equivalent of biologic MIRVs. The antigen-antibody complex, for example, may trip the complement system. Complement release seems an inordinately elaborate way to punch holes in membranes, but in the process it spins off fragments that enlist other responses—chemotaxis of leukocytes, opsonization, and kinin-like activity, to name a few. Platelets adhere; mononuclear cells intrude. The locale may be suffused with lysosomal enzymes, kinins, fragments of complement, superoxide, arachidonate products (prostaglandins, thromboxane), chemotactic factors, and probably other potent factors yet to be elucidated. Somehow order is eventually restored when the danger is past, but the processes of restraint and repair are even less well understood than those of deployment of the defensive arsenal.

Some years ago a senior academician was heard to aver that the only autoimmunity he believed in was that exhibited by a colleague who had miraculously escaped unscathed from three highway accidents. Such skepticism ignores the play of Murphy's law in medicine: "If anything can go wrong, it will." It asks too much that immunity, for example, should be itself immune from error. In fact, host defense not infrequently goes awry, producing diseases that can be crudely defined as those of too much or too little. Disorders of too little defense are simpler to understand in the global or selective vulnerabilities that may ensue in the compromised host. The diseases of too much host defense are more puzzling and more often productive of chronic disability. Mast cells fire off perversely in extrinsic asthma or in the anaphylaxis of insect sting allergy in ways totally inappropriate for the antigen challenge. This excessive cellular xenophobia is clearly injurious to the host. Antigen-antibody complexes fix themselves to glomerular basement membranes, there to incite all the elements of inflammatory injury, rather than being quietly retired from combat by the reticuloendothelial system. Systemic lupus erythematosus has been described as immunological epilepsy because of the vast dissonance that perturbs the immune system in that puzzling disorder. There does seem to be true autoimmunity in Hashimoto's thyroiditis and Goodpasture's syndrome rather than secondary tissue injury in the struggle against some exogenous antigen.

Among the diseases associated with disordered immunity are the vasculitides, which constitute the subject of this monograph. They present as a confusing array of syndromes and overlapping pathologies. By some molecular mischance, immune complexes are formed of a size or possessed of other properties that cause them to adhere to vessel walls. What provokes the formation of these antibodies as the inciting antigen? The discovery that the hepatitis B virus not infrequently fills that role in polyarteritis nodosa is of extraordinary interest. After all, this virus was discovered serendipitously in the blood of an Australian aborigine. Perhaps with equal luck and perspicacity analogous agents can be found for the other two thirds of cases of polyarteritis and for other disorders marked by idiopathic vasculitis. In fact, as this monograph relates, some are already known. Why do some immune complexes circulate harmlessly and others precipitate to cause serious injury to the host? How does one recognize the various clinical entities into which the vasculitides have been classified and what do they imply in prognosis? Of particular importance, what is the state of the art in therapy for this group of disorders?

The study of patients with vasculitis has been a major project at the National Institutes of Health for the past 15 years. This sustained effort has resulted in a number of important contributions and a broad clinical experience. In this monograph, *The Vasculitides*, Thomas R. Cupps and Anthony S. Fauci have drawn upon that experience as well as upon the work of others in compiling this scholarly review. Although not all of the answers to the questions posed earlier are in hand, an impressive start has been made. I suspect that this volume will remain the definitive clinical description of the puzzling group of disorders that constitute the vasculitides for many years to come.

LLOYD H. SMITH, JR., M.D.

PREFACE

The clinical spectrum of vasculitis comprises some of the most interesting and yet perplexing groups of diseases in clinical medicine. Since vasculitis is a clinicopathologic process that is ultimately expressed as a number of diverse clinical syndromes and is not a single disease, there exists an extraordinary degree of heterogeneity together with considerable overlap among the syndromes. It is for these reasons that study of the vasculitic syndromes has caused such confusion and dismay to investigators and practicing physicians who have attempted to fully understand these disorders.

We have been intensively studying the vasculitides in a prospective fashion for the past 15 years at the National Institutes of Health. From this study we have drawn much of the material described here and referred to as our personal experience. Most of this information has been reported in series of articles throughout the years. In addition, we have extensively reviewed the literature and have drawn upon these latter studies to develop a comprehensive approach to the syndromes in question. Many of the original and review articles were written at a time when the classification of the vasculitic syndromes was somewhat uncertain. Thus, many writers and reviewers have referred to the same diseases by different names and have grouped together a number of disorders that today would clearly be distinguished. On the other hand, several investigators have separately classified certain diseases that might best be considered within a single group. Thus, it has been extremely difficult to develop a totally consistent pattern from the literature itself. Hence, rather than merely reporting on the large volume of material contained in the literature on this subject, we have critically evaluated many of the original review articles as well as the countless case reports and small series of patients in an attempt to distill the pertinent and, to the best of our knowledge and impressions, accurate material. To this matrix of information we have added our own prospective studies to create what we hope is an accurate and comprehensive picture of this wide spectrum of diseases. To this end, we have approached the subject

from the pathogenic, immunologic, pathologic, clinical, and therapeutic standpoints. This book has been written specifically for practicing physicians, be they in academic centers or in the private
practice of medicine and related disciplines in the community. It is
hoped that the information contained will serve as a guideline for the
intellectual understanding of the clinicopathologic process of vasculitis as well as for the practical approach to the diagnosis and management of patients with vasculitic disorders. This area of clinical
medicine is advancing rapidly, and greater insights into pathogenesis
as well as the development of more precise and specific modalities
of therapy are surely imminent. It is hoped that this book will provide
the reader with a degree of insight into these fascinating groups of
diseases such that future advances can be appreciated and carefully
evaluated in the framework and context of this insight.

THOMAS R. CUPPS, M.D.
ANTHONY S. FAUCI, M.D.

ACKNOWLEDGMENTS

The expert secretarial assistance of Cynthia Earp and Joni Stefanelli is appreciated, and the editorial help of Betty Sylvester and Joan Barnhart is gratefully acknowledged. A special thanks is extended to Candace Cupps for her invaluable assistance in reviewing this manuscript. The patience of our families and close colleagues during the preparation of this manuscript is appreciated.

Finally, we wish to thank Dr. Sheldon M. Wolff and the clinical staff of the National Institute of Allergy and Infectious Diseases for their invaluable assistance in the clinical management of several of the patient populations discussed in this monograph.

CONTENTS

Neurol. Clinics 11/97

CHAPTER 1

CLASSIFICATION OF THE VASCULITIDES

Definition. Vasculitis is a clinicopathologic process characterized by inflammation and necrosis of blood vessels. The clinical spectrum ranges from a primary disease process involving blood vessels exclusively to an involvement of vessels as a relatively insignificant component of another underlying systemic disease.[1]

Since inflammation of blood vessels can potentially involve any vessel in the body, dysfunction of any organ system may be part of a vasculitic process. The resultant potentially complex clinical presentation was, and still is, reflected in a wide variety of confusing terms used to describe vasculitic syndromes. An historical review of the major vasculitic syndromes will help put the current classification scheme into perspective (Table 1–1).

The early classification schemes were based on pathologic parameters such as vessel size (large, medium, or small), location of vessels (aortic arch, pulmonary, abdominal, or cutaneous), kind of vessel (muscular artery, arteriole, venule, vein, or combination), histologic picture, including kind of infiltrate (polymorphonuclear leukocytes, mononuclear, or giant cells), and location of vessel involvement (intima, media, elastic lamina, adventitia, or panarteritis). Further modifications were required as additional information on pathophysiology became available, new laboratory techniques such as angiography were developed, assays for immune complexes were perfected, and new vasculitic syndromes were defined.

The first vasculitic syndrome described, "periarteritis nodosa," would now be classified in the polyarteritis nodosa (PAN) group of systemic necrotizing vasculitis (Table 1–1). In 1866, Kussmaul and Maier[2] used the term "periarteritis nodosa" to describe grossly visible nodules seen along the course of intermediate-sized muscular arteries. Subsequent reports on this vasculitic syndrome (reviewed in reference 4) established the clinical entity that is now considered classic PAN. This disease is characterized by segmental vascular lesions in different stages of evolution along medium-sized muscular arteries, particularly at branching points. Fibrinoid necrosis of blood vessel walls with aneurysm formation ("nodules") is noted. There is a predilection for renal and visceral arteries with sparing of the pulmonary circulation, splenic follicular arterioles, and other small vessels.

Further definition of the PAN group was made with the description of what is currently called allergic angiitis and granulomatosis (Table 1-1). In 1951, Churg and Strauss[3] described a clinical

TABLE 1-1. CLASSIFICATION OF THE VASCULITIDES

   I. Polyarteritis nodosa group of systemic necrotizing vasculitis
      A. Classic polyarteritis nodosa
      B. Allergic angiitis and granulomatosis (Churg-Strauss variant)
      C. Systemic necrotizing vasculitis "overlap syndrome"

  II. Hypersensitivity vasculitis
      A. Serum sickness and serum sickness–like reactions
      B. Henoch-Schönlein purpura
      C. Vasculitis associated with certain connective tissue disorders
      D. Certain cases of essential mixed cryoglobulinemia with vasculitis
      E. Vasculitis associated with other primary disorders

 III. Wegener's granulomatosis

  IV. Lymphomatoid granulomatosis

   V. Giant cell arteritides
      A. Temporal arteritis
      B. Takayasu's arteritis

  VI. Mucocutaneous lymph node syndrome

 VII. Thromboangiitis obliterans (Buerger's disease)

VIII. Behçet's disease

  IX. Central nervous system vasculitis

   X. Vasculitis associated with malignancies
      A. Polyarteritis nodosa associated with hairy cell leukemia
      B. Granulomatous angiitis of the central nervous system associated with Hodgkin's disease
      C. Hypersensitivity vasculitis
      D. Others

  XI. Miscellaneous
      A. Cogan's syndrome
      B. Hypocomplementemic vasculitis
      C. Erythema nodosum
      D. Eales's disease
      E. Erythema elevatum diutinum
      F. Others

syndrome characterized by fever, severe asthma, hypereosinophilia, cardiac failure, renal damage, and peripheral neuropathy. The pattern of vascular damage was similar to that of PAN with segmental fibrinoid necrosis of muscular arteries and, occasionally, aneurysm formation. The clinical syndrome of allergic angiitis and granulomatosis is distinctive for the involvement of the pulmonary arteries as well as vessels of a broad range of types and sizes ranging from medium-sized muscular arteries, as in classic PAN, to postcapillary venules characteristic of the leukocytoclastic vasculitis seen in the "hypersensitivity" vasculitides discussed further on. In addition, there is marked eosinophilia in the inflammatory infiltrate and granuloma formation. Once the two syndromes, classic PAN and allergic angiitis and granulomatosis, were established, it was apparent that some cases included selected components of both entities, leading to the concept of the "overlap syndrome of systemic necrotizing vasculitis." The polyarteritis group of systemic necrotizing vasculitis represents a continuum between classic PAN and allergic angiitis and granulomatosis. The critical concept is that these syndromes are *systemic* necrotizing vasculitides involving multiple organ systems. In general, this group can be easily distinguished from the group of hypersensitivity vasculitides (see further on), in which there is a predominant and, in most cases, an exclusive involvement of the skin, with other organ system involvement generally being a minor portion of the clinicopathologic picture.

Following the initial description of PAN, two developments were important in establishing another large group of vasculitic syndromes currently known as hypersensitivity vasculitis (Table 1–1). The use of (1) sulfonamides or (2) foreign serum protein resulted in a vasculitic syndrome that was initially confused with polyarteritis nodosa (reviewed in reference 4). Zeek et al.[5] in 1948 firmly established hypersensitivity vasculitis as a separate clinicopathologic entity distinct from classic periarteritis nodosa. Hypersensitivity angiitis is characterized by fibrinoid necrosis of small vessels, predominantly postcapillary venules, with a pleomorphic cellular infiltrate in and around the vessel walls. The skin is the major site of involvement; however, other organ systems may also be affected. Although postcapillary venules are primarily involved, lesions may also involve arteries and veins as well as arterioles and venules. There is no predilection for the branching points of arteries, and the lesions tend to be of the same stage. Serum sickness, drug reactions, Henoch-Schönlein purpura, certain cases of essential mixed cryoglobulinemia with vasculitis, and vasculitis associated with certain collagen vascular diseases may be included in this group.[1]

In 1931, Klinger[6] made the first pathologic description of another disease characterized by a necrotizing vasculitis. The disease was firmly established as a distinct clinicopathologic entity by Wegener in 1936.[7, 8] Wegener's granulomatosis is characterized by a granulomatous necrotizing vasculitis of the upper and lower respiratory tract with varying degrees of glomerular renal involvement.[9] Subsequently, a limited form of Wegener's granulomatosis without involvement of the kidney was identified.[10]

Lymphomatoid granulomatosis, a disease with clinical and pathologic similarities to Wegener's granulomatosis, was established as a separate entity by Liebow et al. in 1972.[11] This disease is characterized by angiocentric, angiodestructive vasculitis of the lower respiratory tract with relative sparing of the upper respiratory tract. As will be discussed in Chapter 7, the cellular infiltrate of the vessel wall is atypical and may develop into a frankly lymphoproliferative process; in this regard, the vessel involvement is not a "classic" vasculitis. In comparison with Wegener's granulomatosis, the renal involvement is an interstitial infiltrate rather than a glomerulonephritis. There is a tendency for involvement of the central nervous system and skin.

The giant cell arteritides, temporal arteritis and Takayasu's arteritis, were both described around the turn of the century.[12, 13] The clinical syndrome of temporal arteritis was firmly established by Horton et al.[14] Temporal arteritis is a disease of the elderly with a widely varied presentation from nonspecific malaise to sudden blindness. Temporal or cranial arteritis is, in reality, a systemic disease, and virtually any large or medium-sized artery can be affected. Characteristically, however, branches of the extracranial carotid arteries are involved with a panarteritis. Infiltration with mononuclear cells, giant cell formation, and fragmentation of the internal elastic lamina are classically seen.

Takayasu's arteritis is predominantly a disease of young females. The clinical manifestations range from generalized symptoms of inflammatory disease to localized problems secondary to constricted blood flow to organs or extremities. The disease follows an exacerbating and remitting course. The pathologic findings are similar to those of temporal arteritis, with a panarteritis involving medium-sized and large arteries but with a predilection for the aortic arch and its branches. Histologically, mononuclear cell infiltrates, intimal proliferation, fibrosis, vascularization of the media, and degeneration of the elastic lamina are found.

Other clinical vasculitic syndromes (Table 1–1) have been described and warrant separate consideration. These diseases or groups of diseases include central nervous system vasculitis, vasculitic syndromes related to malignancies, the coronary vasculitic stage of mucocutaneous lymph node syndrome, Buerger's disease, Behçet's syndrome, Cogan's syndrome, erythema nodosum, Eales's disease, hypocomplementemic vasculitis, and others. Each vasculitic syndrome will be discussed fully in subsequent chapters.

Our current knowledge of vasculitis, particularly with regard to pathophysiology, is incomplete. The classification scheme in Table 1–1 will serve as a framework for evaluating new information. Moreover, the outline will provide an approach to the evaluation of a patient with a vasculitic syndrome. Rapid recognition of the various vasculitic syndromes is of great clinical importance to ensure that appropriate treatment, if available, is started before irreversible organ system damage has occurred. Recognition of the benign forms of vasculitis is also important to avoid unwarranted treatment with potentially toxic agents. Undoubtedly, the classification scheme in Table 1–1 will require further modification as additional information on vasculitic syndromes becomes available.

CHAPTER 2

PATHOPHYSIOLOGY OF VASCULITIS

Although multiple mechanisms may be involved in the mediation of vascular inflammation, vascular damage mediated by immune complexes has been studied in the greatest detail. The animal models of the Arthus reaction and serum sickness have provided valuable information on the conditions under which immune complexes can cause vascular inflammation. Two sections of this chapter will be devoted to immune complex–mediated vasculitis. The first will discuss the nature of the immune complexes and the factors necessary for deposition in vessels, and the second will cover the mediation and expression of the inflammatory response following deposition of the immune complexes. The role of cell-mediated immunity, granulomatous reactions, antibodies directed against vessel components, and other potential pathophysiologic mechanisms will also be described in separate sections. Although these mechanisms for vascular damage are discussed individually, any combination of them may be involved in the expression of a vasculitic process. Finally, the role of immunoregulation and immunogenetics will be discussed.

IMMUNE COMPLEXES

The Arthus reaction provided an important animal model of localized immune complex–mediated vascular damage.[15] The classic Arthus reaction was produced by active immunization of an experimental animal with an antigen such as heterologous albumin followed by a cutaneous injection of the same antigen (Fig. 2–1). In other words, antigen was injected into the skin of an animal with circulating specific antibody against the injected antigen. A local lesion was

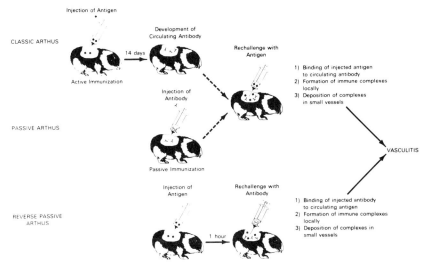

Figure 2–1. Classification of the Arthus reaction. In the *classic Arthus reaction,* the experimental animal is immunized with a specific antigen and produces antibodies against this antigen. Local rechallenge with the same antigen results in *in situ* immune complex formation in the vessel wall and progression to vasculitis. In the *passive Arthus reaction,* antibody directed against a specific antigen is injected followed by a challenge with the specific antigen, which results in local formation of immune complexes in the vessel wall and progression to vasculitis. In the *reverse passive Arthus reaction,* injection of a specific antigen followed by a local injection of antibody against this specific antigen results in immune complex formation in the vessel wall and subsequent progression to vasculitis.

characterized by increased vascular permeability, edema, and polymorphonuclear leukocyte (PMN) infiltration of the postcapillary venules, followed by hemorrhagic necrosis. Similar lesions could be produced in an unimmunized animal by passive immunization with systemic injections of immune serum followed by local injection of antigen. Conversely, systemic injection of antigen and local injection of immune serum also produced the vascular lesions. In the early lesions of these three kinds of Arthus reactions (classic, passive, and reverse passive), antibody and antigen could be demonstrated by immunofluorescence in the vessel wall. These observations demonstrated that *in situ* precipitation of antigen and antibody to form immunoreactive complexes is a potential mechanism of vascular inflammation.

Serum sickness reactions provided a second important animal model for studying immune complex–mediated vascular damage.[16, 17] The syndrome was initiated in experimental animals by injection of a heterologous serum protein such as albumin in a single dose or several closely spaced doses. Over a period of 8 to 14 days the animals developed a syndrome consisting of arthritis, glomerulonephritis, inflammation of the endocardium, and vasculitis. The vascular lesions were particularly prominent in the coronary arteries and branching points of the aorta. Histologically, the lesions began with endothelial swelling followed by an infiltration of PMNs; after 24 hours, infiltration of mononuclear cells was seen.

Studies of the rate of clearance of foreign protein and the host antibody response to the protein provide important clues to the pathogenesis of this model. Initially, there is a phase of slow clearance of antigenic material followed by a more rapid decrease in serum levels. This rapid clearance phase is associated with the onset of clinical symptoms and complement consumption. Finally, antibodies directed against the heterologous protein are detectable in the animal's serum. Immunofluorescent studies demonstrate antigen, antibody, and complement in the early vascular and glomerular lesions. The syndrome of serum sickness could also be produced by intravenous administration of preformed soluble immune complexes.[18, 19] The immune complexes did not demonstrate an affinity for vascular structures.[18] The model of serum sickness clearly demonstrates that deposition of preformed circulating antigen and antibody complexes may be another important mechanism for immune-mediated vascular damage. The mechanisms of circulating immune complex–mediated vasculitis are summarized in Figure 2–2.

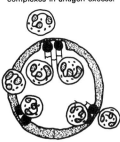
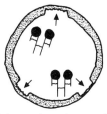
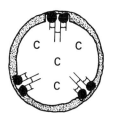

1) Circulating soluble immune complexes in antigen excess.

2) Increased vascular permeability via platelet derived vasoactive amines and IgE mediated reactions.

3) Trapping of immune complexes along basement membrane of vessel wall and activation of complement components (C).

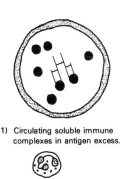
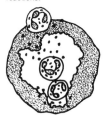
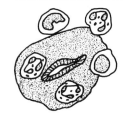

4) Complement derived chemotactic factors (C3a, C5a, C567) cause accumulation of PMNs.

5) PMNs release lysosomal enzymes (collagenase, elastase)

6) Damage and necrosis of vessel wall, thrombosis, occlusion, hemorrhage.

Figure 2–2. Mechanisms of immune complex–mediated vasculitis. Soluble immune complexes formed in antigen excess circulate and are deposited in vessel walls at sites of increased vascular permeability. The increased vascular permeability results from the action of vasoactive amines that are derived from platelets and IgE-triggered reactions. The immune complexes are trapped and complement components are activated, some of which are chemotactic for polymorphonuclear leukocytes which then migrate in and around involved blood vessels. The cells then release their lysosomal enzymes that damage the blood vessel wall. (Reproduced with permission from Fauci AS, et al.: The spectrum of vasculitis. Ann Intern Med 89:660, 1978.)

The characteristics of the circulating immune complexes associated with the animal model of serum sickness were further delineated. Size of the complexes was of particular importance.[20] Only animals with immune complexes with a sedimentation coefficient greater than 19S developed serum sickness.[18] The localization of immune complexes in vessels was independent of both the total electrical charge on the complex and the activation of complement. Studies utilizing skin reactivity in the guinea pig as a marker of biologic activity demonstrated that complexes formed in conditions of slight antigen excess were optimal for deposition.[21, 22] Complexes consisting of a single antibody molecule and a single antigen molecule were inactive. Complexes with two antibody molecules and three antigen molecules had slight activity, but the larger aggregates were even more efficient in producing tissue damage. Finally, there was an association between biologic activity as measured by skin reactivity and the ability of preformed immune complexes to fix complement.

Further evaluation of immune complex deposition included an evaluation of contributory factors at the level of the vessel. Cochrane,[23] utilizing shock induction in guinea pigs, demonstrated that increased vascular permeability was an important requirement for the deposition of immune complexes in blood vessel walls. The increased vascular permeability in this particular animal model was mediated at least in part by histamine.[24] Indeed, vasoactive amines such as histamine or serotonin can promote vascular deposition of immune complexes, while antihistamines and serotonin antagonists are capable of preventing the vascular lesions in certain animal models of serum sickness.[16, 25] Moreover, with the use of colloidal carbon as a marker in these studies, macromolecules could be demonstrated to pass between endothelial cells during periods of increased vascular permeability.[26] The complex molecules (colloidal carbon or immune complexes) were deposited on the luminal side of the elastic lamella of the vessel wall. This concept of passive filtering of immune complexes by the elastic lamella was further defined by Cochrane.[27] Immune complexes greater than 19S in size would remain in the vessel wall. Simple IgG or IgM molecules would pass through the vessel wall but larger complexes, such as heat-aggregated immunoglobulins, would remain. These observations provide a basis for the potential importance of size of immune complexes in the pathophysiology of vascular inflammation.

The mechanisms of increased vascular permeability have been reviewed in detail.[17] The most completely studied model is histamine release from rabbit platelets in which at least four mechanisms have been identified: (1) Soluble immune complexes that lack antibody specificity for platelet antigen will adhere to platelets, causing clumping and activation of the complement cascade. The terminal complement components are involved with subsequent lysis of platelets and release of vasoactive amines.[28-30] (2) Immunologic activation of platelets using a particulate antigen has been demonstrated. Zymosan or erythrocytes, together with antibody to their respective surface determinants, and complement components C1 through C3 will cause clumping of platelets with release of histamine and serotonin. (3) Immune complexes in the presence of C6-deficient plasma and small numbers of PMN will also cause platelet clumping with release of vasoactive amines without lysis.[31] (4) Leukocyte-dependent histamine release has also been described and is mediated by sensitized basophils.[32] Basophils in the presence of IgE and an appropriate antigen will degranulate with the release of histamine and platelet-activating factor. This soluble mediator causes platelets to clump with release of vasoactive amines in an energy-dependent process. This latter mechanism is independent of complement activity. Degranulation of mast cells has also been implicated as a source for vasoactive amines.[24, 33] It is of particular interest that IgE-mediated reactions can participate in the ultimate expression of tissue damage associated with the deposition of immune complexes composed of antigen and antibodies of other Ig classes. Thus, there clearly is a potential overlap and even synergy between immediate hypersensitivity (IgE-mediated) and immune complex–mediated immunopathologic phenomena.

Mechanical factors at the level of the vessel have also been implicated in the pathogenesis of immune complex–mediated vascular damage. The increased frequency of serum sickness lesions at the branching points of vessels suggests that turbulent flow may be a contributory factor. In this regard, hypertension increased the severity and frequency of the vascular lesions in animal models of serum sickness.[34] In the rabbit model, depletion of platelets (a major source of histamine) prevented the lesions at the branching points.[25] The deposition of platelets in areas of turbulent flow may predispose to localization of immune complexes by the release of vasoactive amines and resulting increase in vascular permeability, as discussed earlier. Areas of high shear stress, such as the aortic arch or surgically produced coarctations, developed vascular lesions despite platelet depletion.[25] This finding suggests that if the shear force is sufficiently severe, mechanical interruption of the vascular endothelium may provide an alternative predisposition toward immune complex deposition. Finally, the lesions of hypersensitivity vasculitis are much more prominent in the lower extremities and other dependent areas, such as the sacrum in supine patients. Increased hydrostatic pressure may contribute to the development of lesions in the postcapillary venules of the lower extremities.

Another factor, efficiency of clearance of immune complexes by the reticuloendothelial system (RES), may also be extremely important under certain circumstances. Earlier studies on serum sickness using colloidal carbon demonstrated that the majority of these particles were cleared by the RES and that saturation of the RES markedly reduced the dose of colloidal carbon required for localization in vessels.[26] Subsequent studies demonstrated that the RES would rapidly remove by phagocytosis larger antigen-antibody complexes, but smaller complexes were less rapidly cleared.[35] Pretreatment of the animal with immune complexes would also inhibit subsequent clearance of colloidal carbon by the RES. In animal models, saturation of the RES with soluble immune complexes results in a marked delay in clearance of these aggregates.[36] The increase in circulating half-life of the complexes may predispose to deposition at other sites, such as glomeruli or blood vessels. Attempts to demonstrate RES clearance abnormalities in diseases with altered immunity using aggregated albumin have not been particularly productive.[37] Recently, ^{51}Cr-labeled IgG-sensitized autologous erythrocytes have been used to evaluate Fc-receptor–mediated clearance by the RES. Using these targets, markedly delayed clearance times have been demonstrated in patients with active systemic lupus erythematosus[38] and patients with Sjögren's syndrome. It is of particular note that patients with Sjögren's syndrome limited to the exocrine glands had normal RES function, whereas those with widespread extraglandular disease had markedly abnormal RES function.[39] Since both of these diseases may have vasculitis as a major component, the defective RES function could clearly contribute to the deposition of circulating immune complexes in vessel walls. In this regard, it has been reported that reversal of impaired splenic RES function was accomplished by plasma exchanged in a heterogeneous group of patients with nephritis or vasculitis or both.[40] The precise relationship, if any, between integrity of RES function and the expression of the various vasculitic syndromes is currently under investigation (Fauci AS, et al., unpublished observations).

MECHANISM OF TISSUE DAMAGE FOLLOWING IMMUNE COMPLEX DEPOSITION

The complement system is critical in the mediation of the inflammatory response following deposition of immune complexes. By depletion of the complement components beyond C2 by cobra venom factor, the vascular inflammatory lesion in animal models of serum sickness did not develop despite deposition of immune complexes.[41] One of the major roles of complement in the expression of immune complex–mediated tissue damage is the chemoattraction of PMNs to the site of immune complex deposition. Immune complexes are capable of activating the early components of the classic complement pathway, including C3.[42] The activated C3 component can bind to a C3 receptor on the surface of a PMN and "hold" the cell at the site of immune complex deposition by the phenomenon of immune adherence.[43, 44] Moreover, activation of the complement system produces a number of components, particularly C5a, that promote migration of PMNs to the inflammatory site via a chemotactic gradient.[45-47] The precise role of chemotaxis in the lesions of experimental serum sickness is unclear because maintenance of a chemotactic gradient in a vessel with high blood flow would be difficult. Alternatively, these components may contribute to the inflammatory process by causing mast cell degranulation, histamine release, and increased vascular permeability.[46]

Regarding the cellular elements in these processes, PMNs play a major role in the mediation of the inflammatory response in the animal models of immune complex–mediated disease. With depletion of PMNs by administration of nitrogen mustard, the vasculitis of the Arthus reaction and serum sickness model is abolished despite subendothelial deposition of immune complexes.[48-51] The contribution of the PMN to the pathophysiologic mechanisms following deposition of immune complexes is multifaceted. The PMNs migrate into the area of deposition and phagocytose the immune complexes[50] such that within 24 to 48 hours immune complexes are usually no longer detectable in the vascular lesions. Thus, phagocytosis and proteolytic degradation of the immune complexes appear to be of major importance in the clearance of the deposited complexes and resolution of the vasculitis. On the other hand, in addition to phagocytosis, PMN lysosome contents are released into the area of inflammation by a process of exocytosis. The lysosomes contain a variety of enzymes, including hydrolase, proteases, elastase, lipase, and collagenase, which alter or destroy structures in the tissue. During the Arthus reaction the venule basement membrane is structurally and functionally altered during neutrophil invasion.[52] In rabbit PMNs, this activity is mediated by cathepsins D and E,[52] while a similar activity in human PMNs is expressed by a neutral protease.[53] Collagenase may contribute to the basement membrane destruction by augmenting hydrolysis of collagen-like components within the structure.[54] In a similar manner, destruction of the internal elastic lamina in experimental serum sickness is dependent on the presence of PMNs.[51] An elastase found in the PMN lysosome is probably responsible for this activity.[55] The characteristics and potential mechanisms of immune complex vasculitis are summarized in Table 2-1.

The potential role of prostaglandins in this process deserves comment because of their important effects on both platelets and PMNs.[56] Prostaglandins are potent hormones that are oxidation products of polyunsaturated fats. It is interesting to compare sites where prostaglandins may have regulatory significance with the steps previously discussed in immune complex–mediated vasculitis. The role of platelets in the rabbit model of serum sickness has been emphasized. Activated platelets secrete vasoactive mediators, including prostaglandins and prostaglandin derivatives such as thromboxane A_2, which can aggregate platelets.[57] In contrast, vascular endothelium produces a labile prostaglandin, prostacyclin (PGI_2), which inhibits platelet aggregation and appears to be a natural antagonist to thromboxane A_2.[58, 59] It is possible that an imbalance between thromboxane A_2 and prostacyclin at sites of increased vascular stress could explain platelet aggregation in these areas, with the subsequent cascade of events leading to vasculitis in the animal model of serum sickness. This suggested mechanism is highly speculative at best, but further research in this area is clearly warranted.

Prostaglandins may also play a modulating role in the PMN-mediated inflammatory response.[56] Arachidonic acid derivatives can modulate several PMN functions; both facilitation[60, 61] and inhibition[62] of chemotaxis have been reported. By altering the level of intracellular cyclic nucleotides, prostaglandins such as PGE can modulate

TABLE 2-1. *CHARACTERISTICS AND POTENTIAL MECHANISMS OF IMMUNE COMPLEX–MEDIATED VASCULITIS*

QUALITY OR CHARACTERISTIC	POSSIBLE MECHANISM

Circulating soluble immune complexes
  a. Formation in slight antigen excess
  b. > 19S in size
	Faulty immunoregulation with potentially abnormal monocyte, T cell or B cell interactions
	Failure of RES to clear complexes

Deposition of immune complexes below the endothelium
  a. Increased vascular permeability
  b. "Filtration" of complexes by elastic lamina, or basement membrane
	Mechanisms of increased permeability
	  a. Soluble immune complexes adhere to platelets with activation of complement, platelet lysis, and release of vasoactive amines
	  b. Particulate antigen with antibody, early components of complement through C3, platelet adherence followed by release of serotonin and histamine
	  c. Immune complexes, C6-deficient serum, and small numbers of PMNs will cause platelet adhesion and release of vasoactive amines in the absence of platelet lysis
	  d. IgE-sensitized basophils release histamine and platelet-activating factor

Attraction of PMNs to the site of immune complex deposition
  a. Ability to fix complement
	Complement fixation by immune complexes
	  a. Generation of chemoattractants, including C5a
	  b. Immune adherence

Inflammatory response with destruction of vascular structures	Release of proteolytic enzymes Role for prostaglandins in regulation of the inflammatory response

the release of lysosomal contents.[56] Moreover, PMNs, following activation at the cell surface, are capable of generating thromboxane, which may further modulate the inflammatory response.[63] In this regard, treatment with PGE and a stable derivative, 15–(S)–15 methyl PGE_1, markedly suppressed immune complex–mediated vascular damage in an animal model.[64] The prostaglandin does not prevent immune complex deposition or complement activation in the vessel wall, but it appears to inhibit PMN chemotaxis and enzyme secretion functions.

Although the mechanisms of immune-mediated tissue destruction are discussed in separate sections, it is important to emphasize that several mechanisms may be involved in the expression of immune-mediated disease of which vasculitis may be an important component. Lung involvement is an excellent example of the complex nature and interactions of the pathophysiologic mechanisms that may be involved in immune-mediated diseases. Several of these potential mechanisms for immune-mediated disease in the lung are summarized in Figure 2–3. Following antigenic stimulation in the lung, several responses are possible, including local proliferation of lymphoid cells as well as a systemic proliferation of cells. Subsequent reactions may include cell-mediated tissue destruction, lymphoproliferative disease, and antibody production with immune complex formation. Finally, immune complexes may produce disease by causing a vasculitis or producing more direct tissue damage, as seen with

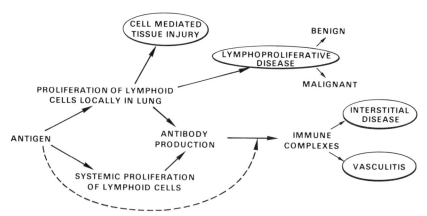

Figure 2–3. Schematic representation of several of the potential mechanisms of immune-mediated lung disease. Reactions to an endogenous or exogenous antigen may lead to triggering and proliferation of lymphoid cells systemically and locally in the lungs. These cells may lead to cell-mediated tissue injury with or without formation of granulomata. They may also proliferate and lead to benign or malignant lymphoproliferative disease in the lung. Furthermore, antibody production and immune complex formation may occur and lead to vasculitis, interstitial lung disease, or both. (Reproduced with permission from Hunninghake GW, Fauci AS: Pulmonary involvement in the collagen vascular diseases. Am Rev Respir Dis *119*:471, 1979.)

interstitial lung disease. It is important to appreciate that multiple mechanisms of immune-mediated tissue destruction may be involved in producing a given pattern of clinical disease.

A causal role for immune complexes has been suggested for a number of the vasculitic syndromes.[1] An association between hepatitis B antigen, immune aggregates consisting of hepatitis B antigen complexed with antibody, and the development of systemic necrotizing vasculitis has been observed.[65, 66] Hepatitis B antigen, IgM, and complement have been demonstrated in vasculitic lesions, suggesting a causative role for immune complexes in systemic vasculitis.[67] Moreover, antigens from streptococcal, staphylococcal, and mycobacterial organisms have been demonstrated in some cutaneous allergic vasculitic lesions.[68, 69] Even rheumatoid factor (IgM anti-IgG-Fc specific) associated with IgG can produce immune complexes that may be involved in the vasculitis associated with rheumatoid arthritis.[70] Failure to demonstrate antigens or immunoglobulins in all lesions is not surprising in light of the technical constraints in identifying various antigens, the probable modification of the antigen within the immune complex, and the rapid clearance of immune complexes as demonstrated in experimental models of vasculitis.[50]

An interesting observation was made by Parish[71] that patients developing vasculitis following a streptococcal infection have decreased antibody responses to M proteins, group A polysaccharide, and streptococcal enzymes prepared from their respective culture isolates when compared with patients infected with streptococcus who did not develop vasculitis. A defect for whatever reason in the antibody response to a given antigen may lead to the formation of immune complexes in antigen excess. Since immune complexes formed under conditions of antigen excess predispose to deposition of circulating complexes in blood vessel walls,[21, 22] it is quite possible that such a deficiency of antibody response could contribute to the immunopathologic mechanisms resulting in immune complex–mediated vasculitis.

GRANULOMATOUS REACTIONS AND VASCULITIS

In contrast to immune complex–mediated vasculitis, other mechanisms of vascular damage are less well studied. The potential mechanisms for granulomatous reactions have been previously discussed.[1] These immune pathways are summarized in Figure 2–4. In a classic type IV reaction, a sensitized lymphocyte reacts with an antigen with release of a variety of mediators. Lymphokines, including macrophage migration inhibitory factor, result in accumulation of activated macrophages. These cells may release their lysosomal enzymes, causing effects similar to the neutrophil-mediated vascular

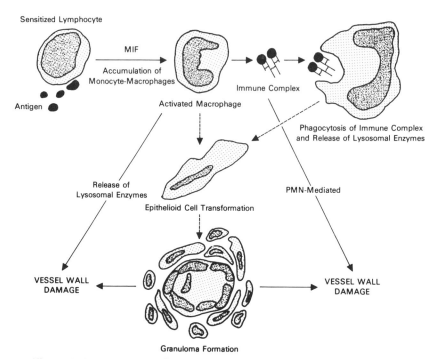

Figure 2–4. Immune mechanisms of granulomatous vasculitis. Sensitized lymphocytes react with antigen and most likely release lymphokines. Some of these soluble products, such as macrophage migration inhibitory factor, result in the recruitment of monocytes to the immune reaction site. These cells may transform into activated macrophages that can release lysosomal enzymes capable of damaging blood vessel walls. In addition, these cells may further transform to epithelioid cells and ultimately participate in granuloma formation. When this takes place in and around blood vessels, granulomatous vasculitis occurs. Furthermore, it is possible that macrophages, under certain circumstances, phagocytose or are triggered by immune complexes. This process may then lead to transformation to epithelioid cells, granuloma formation, or release of lysosomal enzymes. (Reproduced with permission from Fauci AS, et al: The spectrum of vasculitis. Ann Intern Med 89:660, 1978.)

damage. Alternatively, a true granulomatous reaction can develop by transforming monocytes to activated macrophages and subsequently to the epithelioid cells and multinucleated giant cells of classic granulomata.[72]

Furthermore, phagocytosis of certain types of immune complexes by macrophages may result in vascular damage, again by release of lysosomal enzymes or initiation of events leading to a granulomatous reaction. Indeed, antigenic material has been identified in the monocytes in the Arthus vasculitis model.[50] In addition, immune complexes may activate the macrophage by interaction of the Fc portion of the immunoglobulin molecule in the complex and the Fc receptor on the surface of the macrophage. These mechanisms may be responsible for the mononuclear cell infiltration seen in certain types of cutaneous vasculitis,[73] as well as the intravascular and extravascular granulomata characteristically seen in the granulomatous vasculitides.[74] Moreover, the immune complex–mediated granulomatous formation may explain the presence of granulomata in diseases such as allergic angiitis and granulomatosis (see Chapter 4), which also show evidence of immune complex mediation.

DIRECT LYMPHOCYTE-MEDIATED VASCULAR DAMAGE

The role of direct cell-mediated immunity in clinical and animal models of vasculitis is poorly defined. Biopsies of delayed hypersensitivity skin lesions show perivascular accumulation of mononuclear cells, suggesting a potential for lymphocyte-mediated inflammation to involve vascular tissue. Moreover, the presence of granulomata in several vasculitic syndromes, as discussed in the previous section, again points to a role for cell-mediated immunity. In addition, there are several mechanisms of cell-mediated cytotoxicity that could be of theoretical importance. Antibody-dependent cellular cytotoxicity involves the destruction of sensitized target cells through the interaction of the target-specific antibody with effector cell surface Fc receptors.[75] This activity can be expressed by Fc receptor–bearing monocytes, PMNs, eosinophils, and T and non-T, non-B lymphocytes. A second mechanism involves natural killer cells.[76] These mononuclear cells can mediate direct cytotoxicity against nucleated target cells. Neither of these potential mechanisms of cytotoxicity has been evaluated in relation to vasculitis and both are of only theoretical importance at present.

DIRECT ANTIBODY-MEDIATED VASCULAR DAMAGE

Antibody directed against vascular determinants is another potential mechanism of immune-mediated destruction of vessels. This mechanism of autoimmunity is best documented in Goodpasture's syndrome, in which antibodies directed against glomerular basement membranes result in a clinical syndrome of acute glomerulonephritis and pulmonary hemorrhage.[77] Antibodies directed against various components of blood vessels have been produced in rabbits.[78] Intradermal injection of these preparations in humans, however, failed to produce vasculitis. Antibodies to blood vessel basement membranes produced increased vascular permeability.[79] This antibody in the presence of complement and PMNs resulted in destruction of the functional integrity of the basement membrane. A preliminary demonstration of an anti–blood vessel activity in serum of patients with anaphylactoid purpura and polyarteritis nodosa[80] was not substantiated by subsequent observers.[81, 82] There is no compelling evidence to suggest that antibodies directed against vascular antigens play a major role in any vasculitic syndrome.

ROLE OF ALTERED IMMUNOREGULATION IN THE PATHOGENESIS OF VASCULITIS

The preceding sections have discussed the potential mechanisms of immune-mediated destruction of vessels. Perhaps even more important are the immunoregulatory events[83] that result in an inappropriate inflammatory response in the vessel. For example, in patients with systemic necrotizing vasculitis associated with chronic hepatitis B antigenemia,[65, 67] it is quite possible that abnormal immunoregulatory mechanisms prevent the host from making an appropriate antibody response and clearing the viral antigen. Instead, in these individuals a state of antigen excess persists which may predispose to immune complex production and vascular deposition.

Immunoregulatory aberrations have been demonstrated in systemic lupus erythematosus.[84] This disease is characterized by C cell hyperreactivity and a marked decrease in lymphocyte suppressor cell activity. Evaluation of immunoregulatory events in patients with primary vasculitic syndromes is currently under way in our laboratory. In addition to systemic immunoregulation, lymphocytes may modulate activity at the level of the vascular lesion through the release of lymphokines.

The immunoregulatory role of the monocyte also deserves comment. The monocyte is involved in the "afferent" limb of the immune response by antigen processing or presentation.[85, 86] This activity is important in both cellular and humoral immune responses. In addition, the monocyte is involved in the effector limb or the expression of cell-mediated immunity. Furthermore, recent evidence suggests an immunoregulatory role for monocytes in antibody production[87] as well as in cell-mediated immunity.[88] Obviously, any cell with such multiple immunoregulatory functions could be implicated in an aberrant host immune response such as vasculitis. For example, could it be possible that altered antigen processing or faulty B cell regulation by monocytes results in the condition of slight antigen excess that predisposes to vascular immune complex deposition? Although theoretical, such a possibility warrants further investigation.

OTHER CONSIDERATIONS

Another potential mechanism for vascular inflammation is invasion by neoplastic cells. This process is clearly seen in diseases such as lymphomatoid granulomatosis.[11] The angiocentric, angiodestructive vasculitic infiltrate includes atypical lymphoid cells, often with mitotic figures. The high incidence of lymphoma in this group of patients suggests an underlying neoplastic potential.

The potential for environmental or toxic factors is suggested in Buerger's disease, in which there is a close association of disease activity with smoking. Genetic markers in the HLA system have been closely linked with immune-mediated diseases. Among the vasculitides, for example, the increased incidence of HLA-B8 in patients with Wegener's granulomatosis suggests that a genetic predisposition to develop certain types of vasculitic diseases may exist.[89]

SUMMARY

Vasculitis may result from one or more of several mechanisms of immune-mediated inflammation, including deposition of immune complexes and cell-mediated and humoral immune responses. Largely derived from animal models, the mechanisms of immune complex–mediated vasculitis are well defined. The characteristics and potential mechanisms include: (1) soluble immune complexes formed under conditions of slight antigen excess with a size greater than 19S, (2) increased vascular permeability with filtration of immune complexes by the elastic lamina in arteries or basement membrane in venules, (3) activation of complement with the subsequent attraction of PMNs to the site of immune complex deposition, and (4) release of proteolytic enzymes by the PMNs with destruction of vascular structures, including the elastic lamina or basement membrane. The immunoregulatory events leading to the condition of slight antigen excess are of potential importance but have not been well defined.

Both immune complex deposition and classic delayed hypersensitivity cell-mediated immune responses may potentially play a role in the development of granulomatous vasculitis. Currently, there are virtually no convincing data on the roles of classic cell-mediated immune responses or antibodies directed against vessel wall antigens in the development of vasculitis in man. Studies delineating the role of altered immunoregulatory phenomena in the development of vasculitis in man are currently being conducted.

CHAPTER 3

LABORATORY STUDIES
AND DIAGNOSTIC
APPROACH

INTRODUCTION

The diagnostic laboratory studies conducted in a patient with suspected or documented vasculitis comprise a broad spectrum, ranging from routine studies indicating nonspecific inflammatory responses or organ-specific dysfunction, to noninvasive roentgenographic studies, to invasive procedures such as angiography or biopsy. In addition, a number of special studies evaluating immunologic function are available. One of the most important aspects of the diagnostic laboratory approach to patients with a vasculitic syndrome is the orderly, stepwise, and logical use of the available tests such that diagnosis can be firmly established and clinical course followed in the most expeditious manner possible. The present chapter will discuss selected laboratory tests and procedures commonly available and employed in the work-up of patients with vasculitic syndromes. Several of these will be considered in more detail under particular vasculitic syndromes in subsequent chapters.

LABORATORY CONSIDERATIONS

White cell count and differential cell count. In the majority of patients with vasculitis, a mild to moderate leukocytosis is generally present. In addition, superimposition of an infection on the underlying disease, such as a bacterial sinusitis or a lung abscess in Wegener's granulomatosis, may be reflected in a leukocytosis. Leukopenia is

20

unusual in the untreated disease but may be present in patients with lymphomatoid granulomatosis or in those with systemic necrotizing vasculitis associated with hairy cell leukemia. An increased number of circulating eosinophils may be seen with any vasculitic syndrome but is characteristically present in allergic angiitis and granulomatosis.

Anemia. Anemia, if present, tends to be the normochromic, normocytic pattern seen in chronic disease. This pattern seems to be particularly prominent in patients with temporal arteritis. Anemia secondary to external blood loss may be superimposed on the anemia of chronic disease. Blood losses into the gastrointestinal or urinary tract should obviously be aggressively investigated.

Erythrocyte sedimentation rate (ESR). The ESR is a useful tool if its limitations are fully realized. It may be elevated in a wide variety of inflammatory, infectious, or neoplastic processes and therefore lacks specificity. The ESR is generally elevated in the systemic vasculitides. Marked elevation of the Westergren ESR may be seen in patients with either Wegener's granulomatosis or temporal arteritis. Among the vasculitic syndromes, the ESR in these two conditions tends to most accurately reflect the disease activity if other causes of an elevated ESR are carefully excluded. In this regard, the most common cause of an elevated ESR in a patient with Wegener's granulomatosis in clinical remission on immunosuppressive therapy is a bacterial sinusitis rather than a reactivation of the underlying disease. Vasculitic diseases in which the ESR may be normal despite marked disease activity include Henoch-Schönlein purpura, lymphomatoid granulomatosis, central nervous system (CNS) vasculitis, and thromboangiitis obliterans.

Quantitative immunoglobulin levels. Elevation of immunoglobulins is frequently seen in the major vasculitic syndromes. Polyclonal elevation of IgG has been described in patients with systemic necrotizing vasculitis, Wegener's granulomatosis, Takayasu's arteritis, temporal arteritis, Behçet's disease, and Cogan's disease. Elevation of IgA is characteristically seen in such diseases as Henoch-Schönlein purpura,[90] Wegener's granulomatosis,[9] and Behçet's disease.

IgE levels have been evaluated in several vasculitic syndromes. Increased IgE levels have been reported in allergic angiitis and granulomatosis[91] and in certain cases of systemic necrotizing vasculitis.[92] Elevated levels of IgE have also been reported in Wegener's granulomatosis[93, 94]; however, this has not been confirmed in all studies.[95] An elevation of the IgE level has been clearly demonstrated in Kawasaki's disease,[96] including the more severe form (infantile polyarteritis nodosa).[97]

Renal function studies. Renal abnormalities may range from mild proteinuria to rapidly progressive renal failure. Clinically significant impairment of renal function is most commonly seen with systemic necrotizing vasculitis or Wegener's granulomatosis. Less commonly, a decrease in glomerular filtration rate can be seen in the hypersensitivity angiitis group. Abnormalities of urinary sediment are more common. Proteinuria, hematuria, and red blood cell casts may be present in systemic necrotizing vasculitis, Wegener's granulomatosis, and the hypersensitivity angiitis group. Evaluation for the presence of an active urinary sediment can be helpful in differentiating diseases with similar clinical presentations; for example, the presence of an active urinary sediment would favor the diagnosis of Wegener's granulomatosis as opposed to lymphomatoid granulomatosis or midline granuloma.

Rheumatoid factor. Classic rheumatoid factor, IgM antibody directed against the Fc portion of an IgG antibody molecule, can be seen in a wide variety of diseases in addition to rheumatoid arthritis.[98-100] Rheumatoid factor can be seen in rheumatic diseases such as systemic lupus erythematosus, scleroderma, or Sjögren's disease; chronic infections including subacute bacterial endocarditis, syphilis, or tuberculosis; and neoplastic diseases such as lymphoreticular neoplasms, multiple myeloma, or Waldenström's disease. Rheumatoid factor may be seen in patients with essentially any of the vasculitic syndromes but is detectable in a minority of patients and generally in a low titer. It should be pointed out, however, that greater than 50 per cent of patients with Wegener's granulomatosis have positive rheumatoid factor in low titer.[9] Low-titer rheumatoid factor lacks specificity and can be seen in a wide variety of diseases that appear to have in common chronic stimulation or activation of the immune system.

Patients with clinical rheumatoid arthritis and high titers of rheumatoid factor are at greatest risk for developing vasculitic complications. The demonstration that IgG rheumatoid factor and low molecular weight IgM are strongly associated with vasculitic complications in rheumatoid arthritis[101] suggests that antigen-antibody complexes may play a pathophysiologic role in selected vasculitic syndromes.

Immune complexes. The presence of circulating immune complexes has been demonstrated in a wide variety of diseases including rheumatic, infectious, and neoplastic diseases.[102] A significant pathophysiologic role for immune complexes (IC) is most firmly established for the systemic necrotizing vasculitis and hypersensitivity angiitis groups. Some of the most compelling evidence for the significant pathophysiologic role of circulating and deposited immune complexes in the vasculitides lies in the studies that have demonstrated hepatitis B surface antigen (HBsAg) within the circulating cryoprecipitate material[66] and in the deposited complexes in involved vessels[67] in certain patients with HBsAg-associated systemic necrotizing vasculitis. Immune complexes have also been reported in other vasculitic diseases such as Wegener's granulomatosis and Behçet's disease, but the pathophysiologic significance is not firmly established.

The technical aspects of the tests used to make the immune complex determination should be taken into consideration. The relative merits of different methods have been reviewed.[102] For example, the methods that incorporate C1q binding activity in the assay will not detect IgA IC, while the Raji cell assay will. Knowledge of this difference is important in evaluating patients with Henoch-Schönlein purpura or Behçet's disease[103] who may have only IgA immune complexes. Disappearance of detectable circulating immune complexes can be seen in patients who are successfully treated for underlying vasculitic disease.

Cryoglobulins. The spectrum of cryoglobulinemia has been reviewed in detail.[104, 105] The presence of cryoglobulinemia *per se* lacks diagnostic specificity. Cryoglobulinemia has been detected in patients with rheumatic, infectious, and neoplastic disease as well as in those with selected vasculitic syndromes. Evaluation of cryoglobulins provides the diagnostic criteria used to define the group of vasculitides associated with cryoglobulinemia and an exogenous antigen (see Chapter 5). The cryoglobulins associated with this vasculitic syndrome are characterized by a type II or mixed pattern, which generally consists of a polyclonal IgG and a monoclonal IgM with rheumatoid factor (anti-Fc portion) activity. Hepatitis B antigen[66] and coccidioidin antigen[106] have been demonstrated in cryoprecipitates in certain patients with the respective infections and vasculitis. However, this has not been true in all cases.[107]

The importance of appropriate handling of specimens in evaluating cryoprecipitates has been noted.[105] Several points should be emphasized. From phlebotomy to the collection of the serum sample, care should be taken to avoid specimen cooling, which may result in the loss of cryoprecipitable material. Ideally, the blood sample should be maintained at a temperature about 37° C until the serum is collected. During the isolation of the cryoprecipitable material at 4° C, monoclonal or type I cryoglobulins may precipitate rapidly within 24 hours. Samples that are negative at the end of 24 hours should be observed for a total of 72 hours because cryoglobulins, particularly those with a type II or mixed pattern, may precipitate after several days.[105] Another point that deserves mention with regard to the handling of specimens is the fact that certain circulating immune complexes contain cryoglobulins; cooling or freezing of specimens before evaluation for immune complexes may lead to a false negative result, since the immune complexes could potentially precipitate out with the cryoprecipitable material and hence be undetected in the supernatant. Finally, if a cryoglobulin is identified, characterization of the constituents is warranted, including defining monoclonal, polyclonal, or mixed patterns. The presence of a monoclonal pattern makes the diagnosis of an underlying neoplastic process more likely.

Angiography.   Angiography is an important diagnostic tool, particularly in the assessment of patients with systemic necrotizing vasculitis. The role of angiography has been evaluated in 17 patients with well-documented systemic necrotizing vasculitis.[108] The patterns observed include saccular aneurysms, fusiform aneurysms, and vessel narrowing. A complete study should include evaluation of renal and celiac artery circulations because abnormalities may present in one site but not the other. A negative angiogram does not exclude the diagnosis of systemic necrotizing vasculitis.[108] Nor does the presence of aneurysms unequivocally establish the diagnosis, as other conditions, including drug abuse, atrial myxoma, Wegener's granulomatosis, thrombotic thrombocytopenia, and endocarditis, may produce a similar pattern (see Table 4–8). Serial studies may be useful in documenting response to therapy in systemic necrotizing vasculitis.

The usefulness of angiography in other vasculitic diseases, including Takayasu's disease and CNS vasculitis, is well established. Narrowing of the arteries that branch from the aortic arch or the abdominal aorta is the characteristic pattern seen in Takayasu's disease. The pattern of involvement of CNS vessels is most commonly multifocal sites of narrowing, although, less frequently, aneurysms can be seen. It is important to emphasize that a normal angiogram does not exclude the diagnosis of CNS vasculitis and that many other diseases can produce vasculitic changes in intracerebral vessels (see Chapter 10).

Tissue diagnosis.   Frequently, in the evaluation of a patient, one must determine the most expeditious means of establishing a tissue diagnosis. In trying to establish the diagnosis of vasculitis, a systematic approach will be more productive: (1) Make use of any previously biopsied tissue for evaluation. Frequently, patients will have had tissue studies done at other institutions, and not infrequently, a re-evaluation of this material will provide useful diagnostic information. Often, surgically removed specimens such as ischemic bowel are incompletely evaluated, but examination of slides from recut blocks may provide a diagnosis of vasculitis. (2) The choice of biopsy site is also important. There are several parameters to consider, including the ease of obtaining the sample, the morbidity of the biopsy procedure, and the diagnostic return. In general, the sites with evidence of ongoing disease activity will have the highest diagnostic return. Conversely, blind biopsies of asymptomatic sites (i.e., testicular or muscle biopsies in systemic necrotizing vasculitis) are low-yield procedures and are not recommended (see Chapter 4). The diagnostic yield at a particular site varies with the disease; for example, lung tissue has the greatest diagnostic return in Wegener's granulomatosis,[9] while biopsy of an ischemic bowel at laparotomy may have a high diagnostic return in the visceral vasculitis associated with rheumatoid arthritis.[109] (3) It is important that an adequate tissue sample be obtained in order to establish a diagnosis. In general, needle biopsy procedures do not provide an adequate tissue sample to evaluate for vasculitis; consequently, open biopsy procedures may be preferable. A limited thoracotomy with open lung biopsy is the preferred procedure to establish the diagnosis of vasculitis in the lung.[9] (4) Establishing a tissue diagnosis may require multiple biopsies or biopsies in multiple sites. If a biopsy does not provide a diagnosis, the adequacy of the sample should be evaluated; then a decision should be made whether to repeat the biopsy or to biopsy an alternative site.

DIAGNOSTIC APPROACH

Because of the special procedures required to establish the diagnosis of vasculitis, one should carefully consider the differential diagnosis in the approach to a patient with a suspected vasculitic syndrome. Vasculitic syndromes are relatively rare, and frequently the nonspecific presentation may make diagnosis difficult. The possibility of an underlying vasculitic process should be considered in the differential diagnosis of the following clinical syndromes: (1) fever without an established cause, (2) multisystem disease, (3) active glomerulonephritis, (4) ischemic symptoms, particularly in a young person, (5) palpable purpura, and (6) mononeuritis multiplex.

Once the diagnosis of vasculitis is established, the extent of involvement needs to be evaluated, particularly if the diagnosis is based on a skin biopsy. For example, a pattern of small vessel vasculitis may be present in a skin biopsy in a patient with a full-blown systemic vasculitic syndrome such as systemic necrotizing vasculitis or Wegener's granulomatosis. Failure to appreciate systemic involvement may result in the withholding of aggressive therapy and the development of major organ system dysfunction. Thus, evaluation of the extent of disease (localized versus systemic) is extremely important in making therapeutic decisions.

Finally, a wide variety of disease processes can be associated with a vasculitic process. When the diagnosis of vasculitis is established, the patient should also be evaluated for associated diseases when appropriate. Many rheumatic diseases, such as systemic lupus erythematosus, rheumatoid arthritis, Sjögren's syndrome, or scleroderma, may be associated with either small or large vessel vasculitic syndromes. A pattern of hypersensitivity vasculitis may be seen with subacute endocarditis, chronic active hepatitis, ulcerative colitis, retroperitoneal fibrosis, primary biliary cirrhosis, Goodpasture's disease, and neoplastic disorders including lymphoma and leukemias.

CHAPTER 4

SYSTEMIC NECROTIZING VASCULITIS OF THE POLYARTERITIS NODOSA GROUP

INTRODUCTION

Systemic necrotizing vasculitis will be considered as a category that includes classic polyarteritis nodosa (PAN) as well as related disorders in which the common denominator is the systemic involvement with the vasculitic process. The broad category will be discussed in three sections (see Table 1–1). The first section will deal with the clinical syndrome of classic PAN, including a brief discussion of the so-called cutaneous polyarteritis nodosa. The second section will cover allergic angiitis and granulomatosis (Churg-Strauss syndrome). Lastly, the third section will discuss the "overlap syndrome," or clinical spectrum of vasculitis, which includes characteristics from both the classic PAN and the allergic angiitis and granulomatosis groups.

CLASSIC POLYARTERITIS NODOSA

Definition.   Classic PAN is a necrotizing vasculitis of small- and medium-sized muscular arteries.[1, 2, 5, 110] The lesions are often segmental, are in different stages of development, and have a predilection for branching points and bifurcations of vessels. Veins are generally spared unless secondarily involved from adjacent arteries. Involvement of renal and visceral arteries with sparing of the pulmonary circulation is characteristic.

Historical perspective. In 1852 von Rokitansky[111] described the first case of this disease. In 1866 Kussmaul and Maier[2] used the term "periarteritis nodosa" to describe grossly visible nodules seen along the course of intermediate-sized muscular arteries. In 1903 Ferrari[112] first used the term "polyarteriitis" to describe the nodules, correctly emphasizing that the lesions resulted from inflammation of all layers of the artery with subsequent aneurysm formation rather than from a true perivascular process. The point was reaffirmed by Dickson,[113] who introduced the word "polyarteritis." Subsequent authors[114] have suggested that the prefix "poly-" is also appropriate because of the multiple vessel involvement. "Polyarteritis nodosa" is the preferred term because it is anatomically more precise. With the publication of several large clinicopathologic series,[5, 110] classic PAN is firmly established as a distinct clinical entity. The historical perspective has been summarized in detail by Zeek.[115]

Pathophysiology. Evidence from several different sources suggests that PAN is mediated by immune complex deposition (see Chapter 2). Animal experiments of immune complex–mediated disease, including the Arthus reaction and the serum sickness models, show striking similarities to polyarteritis. For example, the vascular lesions produced in animals following injection of heterologous serum (serum sickness model) have a predilection for the branching points of muscular arteries and have a histologic picture remarkably similar to that of PAN.[16, 17] The specific requirements for immune complex–mediated damage include (1) immune complexes greater than 19S in size, (2) increased vascular permeability, (3) activation of complement components, and (4) the presence of polymorphonuclear leukocytes in the vessel.

Patient studies also support the significance of immune complexes in the pathophysiology of PAN. A relationship between PAN and hepatitis was noted in 1947 by Paull[116] following vaccination for yellow fever. The association between hepatitis B antigenemia and PAN is now firmly established. Approximately 30 per cent of patients with PAN have the hepatitis B antigen in their serum.[65, 117, 118] Conversely, the presence of chronic hepatitis B antigenemia appears to predispose patients to the development of vasculitis, at least those patients undergoing long-term hemodialysis.[119] The demonstration of circulating immune aggregates composed of hepatitis B surface antigen and antibody directed against this determinant (as well as hepatitis B surface antigen, IgM, and complement components in vascular lesions) strongly supports the hypothesis that immune complexes are involved in the pathogenesis of PAN. It is important to note, however, that hepatitis B antigen and antibody have been demonstrated in vessels in the absence of vasculitis in cases of chronic aggressive hepatitis.[120]

As previously noted, following deposition of immune complexes, activation of complement plays a crucial role in mediating vascular inflammation.[41] Studies on circulating immune complexes containing hepatitis B surface antigen have demonstrated the presence of IgG, IgA, and IgM. These complexes have the ability to activate both the classic and the alternate complement pathways.[121]

Other infectious agents have been associated with vasculitis. Antigens from streptococcal, staphylococcal, and mycobacterial organisms have been demonstrated in vasculitic skin lesions.[67, 68] PAN has also been associated with elevated anti–streptolysin O titers[122] and poststreptococcal glomerulonephritis,[123] suggesting a role for streptococcal antigen in PAN. Acute serous otitis media in adults has been associated with PAN, although a specific infectious agent has not been identified.[124] Onset of PAN during allergic hyposensitization has also been reported.[125]

PAN may be seen with certain collagen vascular diseases that have a high incidence of circulating immune complexes. For example, systemic lupus erythematosus[126] and rheumatoid arthritis[109, 127] have been associated with necrotizing vasculitic syndromes identical to classic PAN. The recent observation linking PAN to hairy cell leukemia suggests that tumor-related antigens in immune complexes may be involved in the mediation of systemic vasculitis.[128]

A role for hypertension has been suggested in PAN. Hypertension in animal models produced lesions similar to those of PAN.[129] Necrotizing vasculitis has been reported in patients with both primary and secondary pulmonary hypertension.[130] Observations in clinical series of PAN[131] suggesting a primary role for hypertension have not been substantiated. In this regard, it is now generally felt that in classic PAN the hypertension results from, rather than causes, the vascular inflammation. Certainly, elevated blood pressure can exacerbate the vasculitis in animal models of serum sickness.[34] The potential mechanisms for this are discussed in Chapter 2.

Incidence and prevalence. It is difficult to establish a true incidence for this disease because of the variability of classification schemes. There have been in excess of 1000 cases reported since this disease entity was first described.[132] It would fall within a category of what is generally considered an uncommon, but not a rare, disease. The mean age at onset is 45 years (Table 4–1), although PAN has been described at both extremes of age. There is a male to female ratio of 2.5 to 1.

Clinical considerations. Nonspecific signs and symptoms are common in PAN. Fever, weight loss, and malaise are seen in over one half the cases (Table 4–1). The presenting signs and symptoms are reviewed in Table 4–2. Again, it is important to emphasize the relatively nonspecific nature of the presenting problems.[140] Relatively vague symptoms, such as weakness, malaise, abdominal pain, extremity pain, and headache, and myalgias, are quite frequent. Less common signs and symptoms of neurologic and joint involvement are

TABLE 4–1. CLINICAL PARAMETERS IN PATIENTS WITH CLASSIC PAN*

CLINICAL PARAMETER	FINDING	NUMBER OF PATIENTS†
General Considerations		
Age (mean)	45 years	198
Sex ratio (male to female)	2.5 to 1	314
	Per cent	
Fever	71	460
Weight loss	54	405
Organ System Involvement		
Kidney renal	70	375
Musculoskeletal system	64	301
Arthritis/arthralgia	53	301
Myalgias	31	238
Hypertension	54	356
Peripheral neuropathy	51	495
Gastrointestinal tract	44	507
Abdominal pain	43	122
Nausea/vomiting	40	30
Cholecystitis	17	64
Bleeding	6	205
Bowel perforation	5	64
Bowel infarction	1.4	140
Skin	43	476
Rash/purpura	30	259
Nodules	15	369
Livedo reticularis	4	194
Cardiac	36	413
Congestive heart failure	12	204
Myocardial infarct	6	64
Pericarditis	4	204
Central nervous system	23	184
Cerebral vascular accident	11	90
Altered mental status	10	90
Seizure	4	90

*Summary of clinical parameters from references 65, 108, 110, 114, 122, and 133–139, which cover 507 patients

†Denotes the total number of patients evaluated for a given clinical parameter

also described. The nonspecific nature of the presentation and the relatively uncommon occurrence of PAN may contribute to the difficulty in establishing the diagnosis. Moreover, there appears to be little correlation between signs or symptoms and actual organ system involvement with documented vasculitis.[141] The frequency of clinical involvement of various organ systems is reviewed in Table 4–1.

KIDNEY. The kidney, the most frequently involved organ, rarely is responsible for symptoms. Laboratory abnormalities of renal function (urea nitrogen, creatinine, or urinary sediment) are present in 70 per cent of cases (Table 4–3). However, at least three pathologic

TABLE 4-2. PRESENTING COMPLAINTS IN PATIENTS WITH
CLASSIC PAN*

PRESENTING COMPLAINT	PER CENT OF PATIENTS
Malaise/weakness	13
Abdominal pain	12
Leg pain	12
Neurologic signs/symptoms	10
Fever	8
Cough	8
Myalgias	5
Peripheral neuropathy	5
Headache	5
Arthritis/arthralgia	4
Skin involvement	4
Painful arms	4
Painful feet	4

*Data are summarized from 220 patients reviewed in reference 140.

processes may underlie these findings.[110] The most frequent autopsy finding is renal vasculitis, which is present in almost one half the cases. This is followed in frequency by hypertensive changes. Glomerulonephritis is present in nearly a quarter of cases. Renal involvement is of obvious clinical importance, since uremia is responsible for almost one half the deaths in patients with PAN (Table 4–4). Rarely, a renal artery aneurysm will rupture.[142, 143] This life-threatening complication presents with flank and abdominal pain followed by signs of

TABLE 4-3. LABORATORY ABNORMALITIES IN PATIENTS
WITH PAN*

LABORATORY ABNORMALITY	PER CENT†	NUMBER OF PATIENTS‡
ESR >20 mm/hour	94	201
Leukocytosis (WBC >10,000 mm³)	74	292
Anemia (hematocrit >35%)	66	337
Thrombocytosis (>400,000/mm³)	53	17
Renal function abnormality	70	375
Proteinuria	64	250
Hematuria	45	103
Casts	34	64
Complement		
Depressed CH_{50}	21	47
Depressed C3	70	10
Depressed C4	30	10
Rheumatoid factor ≧ 1:160	40	72
Immune complexes present	62.5	32
Cryoglobulins present	25	49

*Data summarized from references 65, 108, 114, 118, 122, 133, 137, and 138
†Per cent of patients with a given abnormality
‡Denotes total number of patients evaluated

TABLE 4–4. CAUSE OF DEATH AS DETERMINED BY AUTOPSY
IN CLASSIC PAN*

Cause of Death	Per Cent	Number of Patients†
Renal	45	107
Vasculitis	45	55
Hypertensive changes	33	55
Glomerulonephritis	20	55
Central nervous system	15	107
Cardiac	13	107
Gastrointestinal	12	85
Bowel infarction	13	30
Massive bleed	3	30

*Data summarized from references 110, 133–136, and 139
†Denotes the total number of patients evaluated for a given cause of death

hypovolemia. Diagnostic x-ray studies generally show a mass effect and a poorly functioning kidney on intravenous pyelography. A delay in diagnostic and therapeutic intervention is associated with significant mortality.[143]

MUSCULOSKELETAL SYSTEM. Arthritis, arthralgias, or myalgias are seen in over one half the patients with PAN. In some patients with hepatitis B–related syndromes, hepatitis B surface antigen and depressed complement levels have been found in synovial fluid.[117] Resolution of arthritis in some cases was associated with clearance of detectable hepatitis B surface antigen from peripheral blood. These findings suggest that immune complex deposition may also mediate the joint symptoms in PAN. The presence of myalgias and the frequent presenting complaints of extremity pain (Table 4–3) may be related to the vasculitis in muscles. Vasculitis is present in skeletal muscle in approximately 40 per cent of autopsy cases (Table 4–5).

HYPERTENSION. Elevated blood pressure, present in 54 per cent of cases, may play an important role in the compromise in renal function. Renal changes secondary to hypertension were present in over 30 per cent of autopsy cases in one series.[110] Diffuse renal vasculitis with secondary hyperreninemia and hyperaldosteronism appears to be an important cause of hypertension in patients with PAN.[144] It should be pointed out that in patients with renovascular hypertension resulting from PAN, the hypertension may persist following the subsidence of active vessel inflammation and hence contribute to the chronic deterioration of renal function by nephrosclerosis, despite the inactivity of the underlying PAN.

PERIPHERAL NEUROPATHY. Involvement of the peripheral nerves occurs in one half the cases of PAN. Various patterns have been described. Mixed motor sensory involvement in a pattern of mononeuritis multiplex is most frequently reported. Other patterns, including mononeuritis and sensory, motor, or distal extremity

TABLE 4-5. ORGAN SYSTEM INVOLVEMENT AT AUTOPSY IN
CLASSIC PAN*

ORGAN SYSTEM	PER CENT	NUMBER OF PATIENTS†
Kidney	85	175
Heart	76	176
Liver	62	105
Gastrointestinal tract	51	175
Jejunum	37	30
Ileum	27	30
Mesentery	24	205
Colon	20	30
Duodenum	10	30
Gallbladder	10	30
Rectosigmoid	10	30
Appendix	7	30
Muscle	39	175
Pancreas	35	175
Testes	33	175
Peripheral nerves	32	204
Central nervous system	27	191
Skin	20	175

*Data summarized from references 114 and 133–136
†Denotes number of patients evaluated

"stocking-glove" involvement, have also been noted. The neuropathy may present with paresthesias, dysesthesias, or weakness. Onset may occur concomitantly with the presentation of the systemic syndrome or appear later in the course of the disease. The lesions, frequently distal rather than proximal, appear to result from vasculitis of the vasa nervorum.[136]

ABDOMEN. Involvement of the gastrointestinal tract is present in 44 per cent of PAN patients. Nausea, vomiting, and abdominal pain, including a pattern of pancreatitis, are frequently noted. Unusual clinical manifestations of bowel vasculitis include "intestinal angina."[145] The syndrome consists of postprandial abdominal pain, anorexia, and ultimately weight loss. Characteristically, the pain starts ½ to 1 hour after a meal and lasts a variable length of time. In one series,[145] 2 of 15 patients with this syndrome had documented bowel vasculitis. A clinical picture of malabsorption and steatorrhea has also been described.[146]

In autopsy studies (Table 4–5) the gastrointestinal tract is involved in one half the cases, with no segment of the bowel spared. In one series the gallbladder and appendix were involved in 10 per cent and 7 per cent of the cases, respectively. The diagnosis of PAN has been made following cholecystectomy[147, 148] and appendectomy.[148, 149] Of note, however, is a syndrome of isolated focal arteritis of the appendix.[150] Long-term follow-up of this group did not show evidence of progression to systemic vasculitis. Necrotizing vasculitis limited to the uterus has also been reported.

Other rarer forms of gastrointestinal tract involvement have been described and include gastric ulceration,[152] acute ulcerative enteritis,[153] and ischemic colitis.[154] There is frequent colonic involvement in the systemic vasculitis associated with rheumatoid arthritis.[109] Perforation of the colon is also described in this group of patients.[155]

Rarely, the abdominal disease of PAN may result in life-threatening surgical emergencies. Major abdominal bleeding (gastrointestinal tract or intraperitoneal), bowel perforation, and bowel infarct are seen in 6 per cent, 5 per cent, and 1.4 per cent of patients, respectively. The figure of 1.4 per cent for bowel infarction may be low because some patients in these series had localized diseases. If patients with documented systemic vasculitis are evaluated, the incidence may be closer to 10 to 15 per cent. There is a high mortality associated with these events.[139] Rapid diagnosis and prompt surgical intervention are crucial to a favorable outcome.[156, 157]

SKIN. In clinical series the skin is involved in approximately 40 per cent of cases (Table 4–1), while in autopsy studies the frequency is 20 per cent (Table 4–5). The cutaneous manifestation of PAN is variable, the most common pattern being a nonspecific maculopapular, purpural, or urticarial rash. A more characteristic nodular lesion is present in 15 per cent of cases. The nodules are located in the subcutaneous tissue and tend to be quite painful.[158] The overlying skin may be erythematous, thinned, and glistening. These lesions tend to come in crops lasting from days to months. The lower extremities are the most frequently involved sites. Rarely, the lesions may progress to frank ulceration. The ulcers may have a superficial, punched-out appearance.[159] Livedo reticularis, a reddish-blue net-like mottling of the skin, is found in 40 per cent of cases. Again, the lesions are more common in the extremities. Less common skin lesions include ecchymoses secondary to a ruptured, subcutaneous aneurysm,[158] gangrene,[108, 158] and vasculitis of the nail folds and digital pulp spaces.[108]

HEART. Cardiac involvement is clinically apparent in a third of patients; postmortem evaluation has documented involvement of the heart in two thirds of patients (Tables 4–1 and 4–5). This observation suggests that cardiac involvement is difficult to detect clinically or that it is associated with a poorer prognosis. The most common expression is congestive heart failure, which may result from coronary vasculitis or hypertension or both.[160] Pericarditis unrelated to uremia or myocardial infarction is seen in up to 14 per cent of cases and appears to be related to the primary disease process.[160] Involvement of the cardiac conduction system has also been reported.[161, 162] Nutrient arteries to the conductive tissue seem to be vulnerable to vasculitis. The sinoatrial conduction system is more frequently involved than the atrioventricular conduction system. The development of cardiac arrhythmias, including supraventricular conduction abnormalities, may have poor prognostic implications.[161] A high frequency of coronary artery involvement and sudden death has been noted in the PAN of infancy syndrome,[163] which will be discussed in detail in Chapter 12, *Mucocutaneous Lymph Node Syndrome (Kawasaki's Disease)*.

CENTRAL NERVOUS SYSTEM (CNS). Clinical and autopsy involvement of the CNS is seen in 25 per cent of patients with PAN. More importantly, it is second to renal involvement with regard to fatal complications (Table 4–4). Clinically, the most common presentation is a cerebral vascular accident (11 per cent), followed by altered mental status (10 per cent) and seizure (4 per cent) (Table 4–1); rarely, cranial neuropathies occur.[164] All vessels may be involved,[135] including both the carotid and the vertebral artery distributions as well as the meningeal arteries. Alternatively, the larger intracranial arteries may be spared, with vascular lesions involving primarily intraparenchymal vessels smaller than 200 μ in external diameter.[165]

EYE. Ocular involvement in PAN has also been emphasized (Table 4–6).[164, 166-169] Hypertensive changes are most common, followed by ocular vasculitis. Vasculitis of the retinal artery may present with retinal artery occlusion,[164, 168] retinal artery aneurysm,[167] and optic disk edema or atrophy.[164] Severe vasculitis of the choroidal and ciliary arteries has been reported[166, 169] and may be clinically silent.[165] Usually, however, choroidal involvement can be seen on funduscopic examination. Globular retinal edema secondary to choroidal vasculitis presents as a raised yellow-to-white retinal "nodule" with sharply defined margins.[164, 167] This edema, if widespread, may predispose to retinal detachment.[164, 169] Rarely, chemosis, episcleritis, iritis, uveitis, granulomatous uveitis, keratitis, and corneal ulcers are present with PAN.[164, 165, 168]

PAN of infancy. PAN in infants (less than 1 year of age) has a unique clinicopathologic presentation, but the diagnosis is rarely made ante mortem.[163, 170-172] Clinically, the disease presents with a

TABLE 4–6. *OCULAR MANIFESTATIONS OF CLASSIC PAN**

PATHOLOGY	PER CENT
Hypertensive changes	19
Central artery occlusion	12
Extraocular muscle palsies	12
Retinal detachment	8
Visual field defects	8
Retinal arteritis	4
Eyelid edema	4

*Data summarized from 24 patients with eye involvement are reported in reference 164. Material from autopsy and clinical sources is included.

transient macular exanthem, transient conjunctivitis, prolonged pyrexia, cardiomegaly, and congestive heart failure. Abnormal urinary sediment, chest x-ray, and electrocardiogram support the diagnosis.[164] Mean length of survival after onset of symptoms is less than 1 month.[164] In comparison with the autopsy findings in classic PAN, this disorder is unique for high frequency (90 per cent) of involvement of the coronary arteries, with relative sparing of the vessels in skeletal muscle (5 per cent).[164] This syndrome is most likely identical to the cardiac involvement in infants with the mucocutaneous lymph node syndrome, which is discussed in Chapter 12.

Laboratory. The results of routine laboratory studies in patients with classic PAN are summarized in Table 4–3. Frequently found abnormalities include elevated erythrocyte sedimentation rate (ESR), leukocytosis (usually with the absence of eosinophilia), anemia, thrombocytosis, active urinary sediment, immune complexes, positive rheumatoid factor, and depressed complement components. Tests for antinuclear antibodies are generally negative. Evaluation of cerebrospinal fluid in patients with CNS disease may be entirely normal or show mild elevations in protein and minimal pleocytosis.[135, 164, 165] Joint fluid examination also frequently reveals a nonspecific pattern.[65, 117] No specific laboratory test is diagnostic of PAN, but the pattern suggests a systemic inflammatory disease involving immune complexes and the complement system.

Pathology. Involvement by anatomic sites is summarized in Table 4–5. There is frequent involvement of the kidneys, heart, and abdominal organs. With the exception of the bronchial arteries, the pulmonary vessels are spared in classic PAN. This point is discussed more fully in the section on allergic angiitis and granulomatosis. The predominant vessel involved is the small- to intermediate-sized muscular artery. The vascular lesions are segmental with a predilection for branching and bifurcation points. Arterioles, venules, and veins are generally spared. Involvement of these vessels is rarely seen, and when present is usually the result of extension of the inflammatory lesion from a muscular artery. Granuloma formation is rarely seen but may be present in 6 per cent of cases.[110]

The various stages of the vascular lesions were described in detail by Arkin.[173] The four stages are: (1) degenerative, (2) acute inflammatory, (3) granulation tissue, and (4) histologically healed end-stage or scar tissue. Destruction of the media and internal elastic lamella with aneurysm formation is characteristic. Endothelial proliferation, vessel wall degeneration with fibrinoid necrosis, thrombosis, ischemia, and infarction occur in varying degrees. All stages of lesion evolution may be seen in an individual patient at any given time. These stages closely parallel the development of vascular lesions of animal serum sickness models: (1) endothelial changes with immune complex deposition, (2) acute inflammatory response with PMN infiltration followed by destruction of the internal elastic lamella, (3) subsequent infiltration of mononuclear cells and a pattern of chronic inflammation, and (4) healing with scar tissue. The simultaneous presence of lesions in all stages of evolution suggests a continued or persistent bombardment of vessels with immune complexes as opposed to an isolated burst of circulating and deposited complexes. This reflection of persistent circulatory complexes is compatible with the persistent antigenemia and circulating immune complexes seen in hepatitis B–associated vasculitis.

The healing stage of the vascular lesion has become more clinically relevant, now that the acute inflammatory lesions can be effectively treated with immunosuppressive agents. Obliteration of the vessel lumen with subsequent tissue infarction, despite control of the acute inflammatory lesions by corticosteroids, has been noted,[174] and late mortality from cerebral vascular accidents and myocardial infarction in patients with PAN[139] suggests that vascular damage may have long-term sequelae. In this regard, vascular damage in experimental serum sickness models can produce lesions similar to atherosclerosis if the animals are maintained on a high-cholesterol diet.[175]

Diagnosis and differential diagnosis. Diseases that may be associated with PAN are listed in Table 4–7. Awareness of these associations is clinically important. In a patient presenting with a picture of PAN, evaluation for these associated diseases is important to ensure an appropriate therapeutic approach. Conversely, in a patient with an established diagnosis such as systemic lupus erythematosus or rheumatoid arthritis, vasculitis may occur with life-threatening complications. A history of drug use is an important part of the evaluation because of the association of PAN with parenteral amphetamine use. This drug appears to have a direct toxic effect in animals even after short-term use.[189]

The mainstay of establishing the diagnosis of PAN is the histopathologic demonstration of necrotizing vasculitis of small- and medium-sized arteries in a patient with clinical manifestations compatible with PAN (Figs. 4–1 and 4–2). The tissue diagnosis of systemic necrotizing vasculitis can be made in any of a number of sites. Surgical specimens such as gallbladder may have the characteristic changes. The vessels leading to necrotic or infarcted bowel removed at laparotomy should be closely scrutinized for evidence of vasculitis.

Because of the frequent finding of vasculitis in skeletal muscle in autopsy series, biopsy of this site has been suggested to establish the diagnosis. In muscle biopsies done in attempts to establish the diagnosis of PAN, there was a true positive rate of 35 per cent and a false negative rate of 65 per cent.[190] The most favorable conditions for obtaining positive results were biopsy of muscle at the site of a subcutaneous nodule in a patient who had been symptomatic for less than 6 months or biopsy in a symptomatic muscle group. Empirical muscle biopsies of clinically uninvolved sites are not warranted, and negative biopsy results do not exclude the diagnosis.

The testis has also been suggested as a high-yield biopsy site to establish the diagnosis of PAN.[191] In careful, complete autopsy evaluations, testicular arterial lesions can be seen in 86 per cent of cases. Given the limited tissue sample obtained, the diagnosis could be firmly established in only 20 per cent of patients with PAN who underwent testicular biopsy.[191] In the absence of clinical symptoms, a biopsy does not seem warranted; furthermore, a negative biopsy result does not exclude the diagnosis. Other potential biopsy sites may be productive in certain clinical situations. Rectal mucosal biopsy may have a high yield in patients with rheumatoid arthritis and necrotizing vasculitis. As noted, renal and hepatic involvement is frequent. The potential risk of bleeding at these sites with a closed needle biopsy should be considered, and angiographic evaluation of these organs prior to needle biopsy seems warranted, since risks of complications associated with bleeding from aneurysms are significant.

TABLE 4–7.   DISEASES ASSOCIATED WITH OR CAUSALLY IMPLICATED IN CLASSIC PAN*

TYPE OF DISEASE	REFERENCE
Infection	
Hepatitis B	65, 117, 118
Acute otitis media	124
Streptococcal infection	122, 123
Endocarditis	176
Collagen Vascular/Rheumatic	
Systemic lupus erythematosus	110, 126
Rheumatoid arthritis	109, 127
Sjögren's syndrome	177
Dermatomyositis	178
Scleroderma	179
Essential mixed cryoglobulinemia	180
Relapsing polychondritis	181
Giant cell arteritis	182–184
Other	
Hairy cell leukemia	128
Amphetamine drug abuse	185, 186
Enteritis	153, 187
Allergic hyposensitization therapy	125
Mesenteric arteritis following surgical repair of aortic coarctation	188

*These diseases have been associated with a necrotizing vasculitis similar to that described in classic PAN. Some of the diseases, such as hepatitis B antigenemia, have been causally implicated in classic PAN.

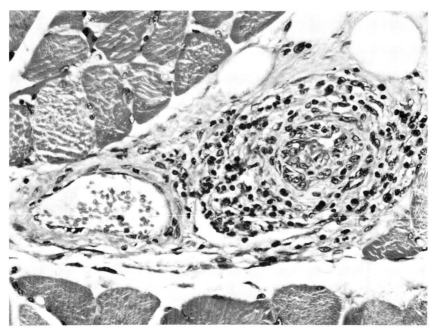

Figure 4–1. Muscle biopsy from a patient with classic polyarteritis nodosa. Necrotizing vasculitis of a small muscular artery with a predominantly mononuclear cell infiltrate is seen. Note the relative noninvolvement of the adjacent vein. Hematoxylin and eosin stain (original magnification ×330).

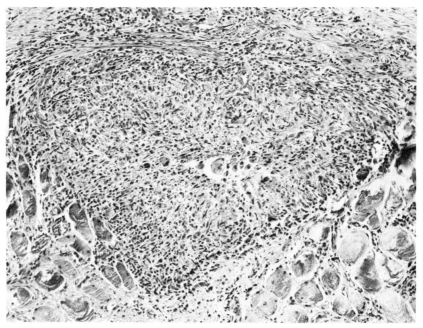

Figure 4–2. Muscle biopsy from a patient with classic polyarteritis nodosa. A necrotizing vasculitis with a mixed cellular infiltrate is seen. There is marked distortion of the vessel wall with near-obliteration of the lumen (original magnification ×130).

Finally, the demonstration of a necrotizing vasculitis at a single site does not necessarily establish the diagnosis of a systemic vasculitis. Vasculitis localized to the appendix[150] and uterus[151] without other systemic involvement has been described. Cutaneous PAN is characterized by necrotizing vasculitis restricted to the subcutaneous tissue or skeletal muscle or both.[192] If tissue from one of these sites demonstrates a vasculitic process, a complete systemic evaluation to determine the extent of involvement is indicated.

Angiographic examination is the second major method of establishing the diagnosis of PAN (Fig. 4–3). The occurrence of multiple intraparenchymal, saccular aneurysms demonstrable by angiography was first reported in PAN on renal angiography.[193] Subsequently, multiple organ involvement[194] and fusiform aneurysms localized in the liver[95] were demonstrated angiographically. The spectrum and importance of angiography in PAN are reviewed in a clinical angiographic analysis of 17 patients with biopsy-proven disease.[108] In this series, an aneurysm was defined as vascular dilatation with a circular appearance; changes in vessel size or caliber were labeled arteriopathy. Undoubtedly, fusiform aneurysms would contribute to the angiographic changes in this latter group. Of the 17 patients studied, 59 per cent had aneurysms, 23 per cent demonstrated arteriopathy alone, and 18 per cent were normal. Aneurysms were found in 60 per cent of hepatic, 47 per cent of renal, and 38 per cent of mesenteric studies, while arteriopathic changes alone were seen in 30 per cent of renal, 20 per cent of hepatic, and 15 per cent of mesenteric artery evaluations. In addition, one patient with abdominal aneurysms also had intracerebral aneurysms. The aneurysms in a given individual tended to be of similar size. The majority ranged in size between 1 and 5 mm, although several aneurysms of between 6 and 12 mm were noted. In all cases, multiple aneurysms were present, and six or more were present in greater than 80 per cent of the vessel groups studied. There was no correlation between clinical evaluation and involvement by angiography of a given organ system.

Angiography will establish the diagnosis of PAN in approximately 80 per cent of patients, but a negative study does not exclude the diagnosis entirely. Angiographic techniques may also be used to identify the source of a bleeding aneurysm. In addition, serial studies can be employed to evaluate the effectiveness of therapy.[196] Although intraparenchymal aneurysms were thought to be diagnostic of PAN, other syndromes may also demonstrate this finding; these diseases are summarized in Table 4–8 and include conditions most likely related to the systemic necrotizing vasculitis group as well as apparently unrelated, distinct entities. In the group of apparently unrelated diseases, patients with a history of drug abuse or with atrial myxomas may present with clinical and angiographic pictures indistinguishable from that of classic PAN. A careful drug use history and a screen for hepatitis B antigen may establish the diagnosis in the former case.

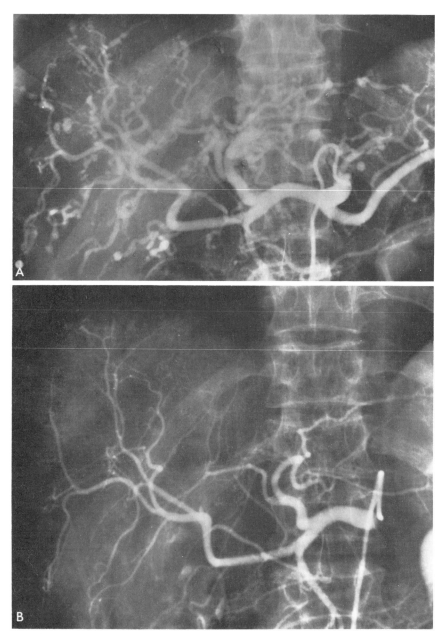

Figure 4–3. A, Hepatic angiogram prior to therapy in a patient with systemic necrotizing vasculitis of the polyarteritis nodosa group. Multiple saccular aneurysms as well as areas of arterial narrowing are seen. B, Hepatic angiogram from the same patient seen in A after 1 year of treatment with cyclophosphamide and alternate-day prednisone. Note the resolution of the multiple aneurysms.

TABLE 4–8. DISEASES OTHER THAN CLASSIC PAN ASSOCIATED WITH ANGIOGRAPHICALLY DEMONSTRABLE ANEURYSMS

DISEASES	REFERENCE
*Related Diseases**°	
Systemic lupus erythematosus	126, 197
Infantile PAN	170
Mucocutaneous lymph node syndrome (Kawasaki disease)	198
Apparently Unrelated Diseases†	
Drug abuse	185
Atrial myxoma	199
Wegener's granulomatosis	200
Thrombotic thrombocytopenia purpura	201
Endocarditis	202, 203
Neurofibromatosis	204
Fibromuscular dysplasia	205
Pseudoxanthoma elasticum	108

°The diseases in this group may be related to the systemic necrotizing vasculitis group.

†The diseases in this group appear to be distinct clinicopathologic entities.

Cardiac ultrasound is the most effective noninvasive technique to diagnose atrial myxomas. The remainder of the diseases in the unrelated disease group are less likely to be confused with PAN. Moreover, in these diseases, angiographic studies usually demonstrate a single aneurysm, which would suggest a diagnosis other than PAN.

Other nonangiographic roentgenographic studies may suggest the diagnosis of PAN. Mesenteric arteritis may cause a pattern of "thumbprinting" on barium contrast studies performed on the bowel. Although intravenous pyelograms are generally normal in PAN, the finding of a retroperitoneal mass effect with an ipsilateral hypofunctioning kidney suggests a bleeding renal aneurysm.[142, 143] Ureteral irregularity with a pattern of partial obstruction may suggest the diagnosis of vasculitis.[206]

Because PAN can involve any organ system, it can be confused with any number of other clinical entities, depending on the mode of presentation. PAN should be considered in the following situations: (1) persistent fever and weight loss in an undiagnosed systemic illness, (2) unexplained cardiac or CNS ischemic events, (3) acute abdomen, (4) active urinary sediment or hypertension or both, (5) myopathy or neuropathy, and (6) skin rash (including palpable purpura, livedo reticularis, and subcutaneous nodules).

Treatment and prognosis. The 5-year survival rate for untreated patients with PAN is 13 per cent.[137] This figure probably includes patients with diseases restricted to the skin and muscle, who have a more favorable prognosis[192]; the true 5-year survival rate for untreated patients with PAN is probably lower. The use of corticosteroids was reported to have improved the 5-year survival rate to 48 per cent.[137] However, although corticosteroids can clearly induce remissions in certain cases of PAN, they frequently induce partial remissions or mask smoldering disease activity so that insidious and relentless organ system damage occurs while a patient is considered to be in an "apparent" remission. This has important implications in that corticosteroids may suppress acute disease activity without substantially affecting the long-term morbidity and mortality.

The use of cytotoxic agents has resulted in major advances in the treatment of PAN.[118, 138] In one retrospective series,[138] the 5-year survival rate increased from 53 per cent for patients treated with corticosteroids alone to 80 per cent for those treated with corticosteroids and immunosuppressive agents. The most commonly used immunosuppressive agents were azathioprine and cyclophosphamide. Cyclophosphamide is clearly effective in inducing clinical remission in patients with severe necrotizing vasculitis who had been refractory to other therapeutic modalities.[118] This drug is effective in controlling far advanced disease in adults[196] and children.[207] No recurrence of the disease has been described in the course of cyclophosphamide therapy,[118] but long-term follow-up of patients in remission and no longer receiving therapy is currently not available in large numbers.

We consider cyclophosphamide the drug of choice in severe, progressive systemic necrotizing vasculitis of the PAN group. Cyclophosphamide is initially administered at 2 mg per kg per day orally together with prednisone, 60 mg orally per day. After 10 to 14 days, the prednisone is gradually tapered to an alternate-day regimen and the cyclophosphamide dose is adjusted to maintain a total white blood cell count of 3000 to 3500/mm^3, which usually results in a neutrophil count of 1000 to 1500/mm^3. Further details of the management of immunosuppressive therapy are discussed in Chapter 15.

Finally, several points concerning general medical management should be emphasized, particularly regarding the careful control of hypertension. Meticulous control of hypertension is warranted for several reasons. Kidneys initially damaged by vasculitis or glomerulonephritis should be protected from additional insult from sustained hypertension. Furthermore, a decrease in late mortality from stroke and myocardial infarction may be appreciated by close control of the blood pressure.

CUTANEOUS POLYARTERITIS NODOSA SYNDROME

Definition. Cutaneous PAN is a disease characterized by a necrotizing vasculitis of small muscular arteries of subcutaneous tissue. The disease is a localized process with sparing of visceral arteries and therefore is *not* a true systemic vasculitic syndrome. Cutaneous PAN runs a chronic course with a good long-term prognosis.[192] Although the histologic lesion resembles that of classic PAN, clinically this disease is similar to the hypersensitivity vasculitis group of diseases (see Chapter 5).

Historical perspective. Case reports describing patients with necrotizing vasculitis identical to classic PAN but limited to vessels in the subcutaneous tissues were the first indications that a disease entity similar in its histopathology to PAN but with limited involvement resulted in a relatively benign course.[208, 209] This clinical entity was finally established by Diaz-Perez and Winkelmann.[192]

Clinical considerations. Although the primary sites of involvement are the skin and muscle, systemic symptoms such as fever and arthralgia are not uncommon. The frequency of skin lesions is as follows: nodular, 83 per cent; livedo reticularis, 78 per cent; and ulcers, 39 per cent.[192] Rarely, the lesions will follow the path of a vessel, and pulsatile lesions have been noted. The lesions are almost uniformly painful and are found most frequently on the lower extremities. An association with inflammatory bowel disease has been described.[187]

Laboratory. Routine laboratory studies generally show a leukocytosis and elevated ESR. Urinalysis and renal function studies are generally normal; electromyography may show a pattern of neuropathy or myositis.[192]

Pathology. The histologic lesion is a necrotizing vasculitis of muscular arteries in the subcutaneous tissue and muscles; the pattern is identical to that seen in classic PAN.

Diagnosis and differential diagnosis. The diagnosis is established by appropriate histologic findings on a skin or muscle biopsy *and* a negative evaluation for systemic involvement.

Treatment and prognosis. Corticosteroids, aspirin, and sulfapyridine have been used with varying success to control the manifestations of the disease. Cases that were clearly refractory to corticosteroids have been noted.[209] We have also certainly seen cases of cutaneous vasculitis unresponsive to prednisone therapy. The use of cytotoxic agents in selected patients has met with a variable clinical response in our experience. However, the dramatic clinical remissions seen in systemic necrotizing vasculitis with the use of cytotoxic agents such as cyclophosphamide have not been observed as consistently in cutaneous PAN. The clinical course is chronic with exacerbations and remissions, and the pain from the skin lesions may be difficult to control. Vasculitis limited to the skin on the initial evaluation does not, as a general rule, progress to systemic involvement. The long-term prognosis even in untreated patients is good.

ALLERGIC ANGIITIS AND GRANULOMATOSIS

Definition. Allergic angiitis and granulomatosis is a disease characterized by a granulomatous vasculitis of multiple organ systems. Although vascular lesions identical to those of classic PAN may be present, this disease is unique for the following reasons: (1) frequency of involvement of pulmonary vessels, (2) vasculitis of blood vessels of various types and sizes (small- and medium-sized muscular arteries, veins, arteries, and venules), (3) intra- and extravascular granuloma formation, (4) eosinophilic tissue infiltrates, and (5) association with severe asthma and peripheral eosinophilia.

Historical perspective. Following the initial report of classic PAN by Kussmaul and Maier,[2] several authors reported cases with vascular lesions similar to those of PAN but with involvement of the pulmonary artery.[112, 113] Ophüls[210] emphasized the presence of eosinophils and granuloma in the pulmonary vasculitis, and the clinical presentation of asthma and peripheral eosinophilia was firmly established.[211, 212] The clinicopathologic parameters that define allergic angiitis and granulomatosis were established by Churg and Strauss.[3] The relationship to PAN was subsequently explored by Rose and Spencer.[110]

Pathophysiology. The presumptive mechanisms of vasculitis are similar in classic PAN and allergic angiitis and granulomatosis. The relationship between immune complexes and apparent expression of atopy (asthma, eosinophilia, and elevated IgE) in this group of patients is unclear. Clinically apparent asthma generally precedes the vasculitis, which may appear as the asthma becomes more severe and intractable, or less frequently may present as the asthma is resolving.[3, 91]

Incidence and prevalence. Allergic angiitis and granulomatosis is a rare disease, but its true incidence is difficult to define. In one series,[81] allergic angiitis and granulomatosis constituted approximately 30 per cent of the overall group of systemic necrotizing vasculitis. The mean age of onset of systemic symptoms is 44 years. There is a male to female ratio of 1.3 to 1 (Table 4–9).

Clinical considerations. There are many similarities in the expression of clinical signs and symptoms in both classic PAN and allergic angiitis and granulomatosis. The spectrum of clinical involvement is summarized in Table 4–9. Of note is the high frequency of pulmonary findings and the less frequent involvement of the kidneys and CNS when compared with classic PAN.

LUNG. Pulmonary signs or symptoms are seen in almost all patients. Asthma and transient pulmonary infiltrates are frequently described. Symptoms related to the lung generally precede evidence of systemic involvement by approximately 2 years, although the range is from 0 to 30 years. Initial onset of wheezing has not been reported

TABLE 4–9. CLINICAL PARAMETERS IN ALLERGIC ANGIITIS AND GRANULOMATOSIS

Category	Results	Number of Patients°
General Considerations		
Age (mean)	44 years	57
Sex ratio (male to female)	1.3 to 1	57
Fever	Majority of patients	–
Duration (mean) of pulmonary symptoms prior to systemic symptoms	2 years	45
Organ System Involvement	*Per Cent*	
Pulmonary	96	47
Infiltrate on chest x-ray	93	47
Wheezing	82	47
Cutaneous	67	43
Purpura	37	43
Nodule	35	43
Peripheral neuropathy	63	43
Hypertension	54	13
Gastrointestinal	42	43
Cardiac	38	13
Renal	38	75
Lower urinary tract	10	30
Arthritis/arthralgia	21	43

°Number of patients for whom the observation was made. The data were summarized from references 3, 91, and 110.

to follow onset of systemic disease, and a shorter duration of pulmonary symptoms has been associated with a poorer prognosis.[91]

SKIN. Cutaneous involvement is present in 67 per cent of cases. Purpura and nodular lesions are found with equal frequency. Livedo reticularis is apparently rarer in allergic angiitis and granulomatosis than in classic PAN. Biopsy of the purpuric lesions reveals typical leukocytoclastic venulitis, which is characteristic of hypersensitivity vasculitis but is not generally seen in classic PAN. Biopsy of the nodular lesions, however, may demonstrate extravascular granuloma with eosinophilic infiltrates[3] as opposed to the true vasculitis seen frequently with PAN.

PERIPHERAL NEUROPATHY. The pattern is similar to that of PAN, with mononeuritis multiplex being most commonly described.

GASTROINTESTINAL TRACT. The gastrointestinal tract is involved in approximately 40 per cent of cases. Gastric ulcers, granuloma of the omentum, small bowel perforation, ulcerative colitis, and inflammatory masses in the colon have been noted.[91] In one series[3] a high frequency of bloody diarrhea was reported. Compared with classic PAN there is a lower incidence of life-threatening intra-abdominal bleeding, probably reflecting the decreased frequency of aneurysm formation seen in this disease.

CARDIOVASCULAR SYSTEM. Clinically, the heart is involved in approximately a third of cases, which is similar to the incidence in classic PAN. Heart involvement at autopsy is 62 per cent (Table 4–10) which again parallels the findings in classic PAN. In addition to the vasculitis of the coronary arteries, nodular pericarditis with granuloma formation, endothelial fibrosis, and eosinophilic infiltrates are described.[3] Elevated blood pressures are seen in approximately one half the cases.

URINARY TRACT. Clinical evidence of renal involvement is half as frequent (33 per cent) in allergic angiitis and granulomatosis as in classic PAN. In addition to the vasculitis, glomerulonephritis, and hypertensive changes, an interstitial infiltrate with eosinophils is described.[3] A high frequency of lower urinary tract involvement, particularly of the prostate, was noted in one series.[91]

Laboratory. Laboratory findings are similar to those found in PAN. An elevated ESR and leukocytosis are found in the majority of cases. An elevated total eosinophil count (greater than $1000/mm^3$) is noted at some point in the patient's course in approximately 85 per cent of cases.[3, 91, 110] Marked variability in eosinophil counts of an individual patient is common. Elevation of IgE has also been described.[91]

Pathology. The anatomic sites involved in autopsy studies are summarized in Table 4–10. The frequent involvement of the spleen and pulmonary vessels with sparing of the CNS is in contrast to classic PAN. The causes of death as defined at autopsy are summarized in Table 4–11. Of note, cardiopulmonary complications account for one half the deaths. In contrast, renal disease and complications from hypertension account for the majority of deaths in classic PAN.

TABLE 4–10. SITES OF VASCULITIS AT AUTOPSY IN ALLERGIC ANGIITIS AND GRANULOMATOSIS

ORGAN SYSTEM	PER CENT	NUMBER OF PATIENTS[°]
Spleen	67	9
Renal (vasculitis)	63	40
Eosinophil interstitial infiltrate	60	30
Cardiac	62	39
Hepatic	48	39
Pulmonary	46	39
Gastrointestinal	33	70
Musculoskeletal	20	39
Central nervous system	3	30

°Number of patients for whom the observation was made. The data were summarized from references 3, 91, and 110. Of note, the skin was not routinely evaluated during the postmortem evaluation. Clinically, skin involvement with vasculitis is frequently seen.

TABLE 4-11. CAUSES OF DEATH AS DETERMINED BY AUTOPSY IN ALLERGIC ANGIITIS AND GRANULOMATOSIS

ORGAN SYSTEM	PER CENT	NUMBER OF PATIENTS[°]
Pulmonary	26	57
Pneumonia	14	57
Status asthmaticus	8	20
Cardiac	23	57
Renal	18	57
Vasculitis	7	
Glomerulonephritis	7	
Hypertensive changes	4	
Gastrointestinal	7	57
Central nervous system (hemorrhage)	5	57

[°]Number of patients for whom the observation was made. The data were summarized from references 3, 91, and 110.

In addition to the segmental lesions of small- and intermediate-sized muscular arteries, involvement of smaller vessels is common (Fig. 4–4). Vessels less than 500 μ in external diameter are frequently involved.[110] Eosinophils and granulomata are seen in and around the vascular infiltrates.[3, 110] The veins are involved in approximately 50 per cent of cases,[3] and venulitis characterizes the purpuric skin lesions. Fibrinoid necrosis, thrombosis, infarction, and aneurysm formation are less frequently noted. Extravascular granulomata are frequently found, particularly in the epicardium and skin.[3] In fact, granulomata with eosinophilic infiltrates are the most common histologic finding in the nodular skin lesion, with vasculitis being less frequent.

Diagnosis and differential diagnosis. There are no prospective studies to define diagnostic yield from a specific biopsy site. Major potential sites include lung and muscle tissue. As with virtually all of the vasculitides, biopsy of sites with evidence of clinical involvement would most likely have the highest return. Radiographic examination may provide important information. However, the role of angiography in establishing the diagnosis of allergic angiitis and granulomatosis is not clearly defined. In this regard, aneurysms have been described angiographically in this syndrome,[108] but the frequency of this finding is unclear at the present time. Abnormal chest x-ray studies are reported in most patients. The most common finding is transient infiltrates lasting from weeks to months.[91] Consolidation is frequent, and there is equal involvement of the upper and lower lung fields.[110] The lesions may have a nodular appearance with an irregular outline.[91, 110] Signs of congestive heart failure, cavitary lesions, interstitial patterns, and pleural effusion are less commonly seen.

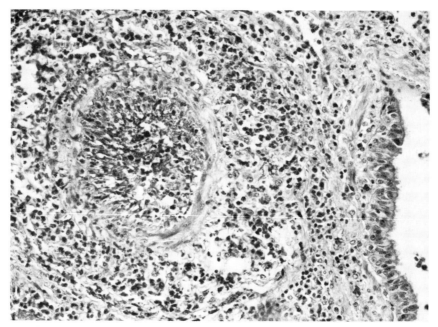

Figure 4-4. Lung biopsy from a patient with allergic angiitis and granulomatosis. A necrotizing vasculitis is seen with an infiltrate composed of mononuclear cells and eosinophils that virtually obliterates the vessel lumen. Multinucleated giant cells were present elsewhere on the slide. Hematoxylin and eosin stain (original magnification × 220).

In addition to classic PAN, diseases associated with granulomata, hypereosinophilia, and cardiac or pulmonary symptoms should be included in the differential diagnosis of allergic angiitis and granulomatosis. Certainly Wegener's granulomatosis, allergic aspergillosis, pulmonary infiltrates with eosinophilia syndrome, sarcoidosis, and the idiopathic hypereosinophilic syndrome could be confused with allergic angiitis and granulomatosis. Although wheezing may abate with the onset of systemic symptoms, some patients may progress to refractory status asthmaticus. Allergic angiitis and granulomatosis should be considered in the differential diagnosis in any patient presenting with refractory bronchospasm and pulmonary infiltrates.

Treatment and prognosis. Although less well documented, the response to corticosteroids and immunosuppressive agents in allergic angiitis and granulomatosis is similar to that seen in classic PAN. Untreated, the disease has a 5-year survival rate of 4 per cent.[110] With the use of corticosteroids, the 5-year survival rate is approximately 60 per cent. The response to immunosuppressive agents has not been studied in detail. Clinical remissions with the use of azathioprine have been reported,[91, 213] but complete remission was not obtained in every case.[213] We have reported a number of complete remissions in this disease with the use of cyclophosphamide, similar to its efficacy in classic PAN.[118]

"OVERLAP SYNDROME" OF SYSTEMIC NECROTIZING VASCULITIS

The third disorder of the group of systemic necrotizing vasculitides is the "overlap syndrome." There are patients who share clinical and pathologic features characteristic of both classic PAN and allergic angiitis and granulomatosis but do not fit precisely into either category. This group has multisystem involvement with the associated protean clinical manifestations. Lesions of muscular arteries may be present, and involvement of arterioles and venules is also seen. The recognition of an overlap syndrome emphasizes that there is a continuum of disease manifestations between classic PAN and allergic angiitis and granulomatosis.

The difficulties in classification have been recently exemplified in a series of patients with hepatitis B and systemic vasculitis.[65] Despite an apparently common causative antigen, there was a wide spectrum of clinical vasculitic syndromes ranging from classic PAN to small vessel vasculitis, in addition to cases that did not fit into a well-defined syndrome. In a similar manner, a wide spectrum of clinical disease was seen in the vasculitis associated with acute serous otitis media.[124] The reasons for the marked variability in clinical presentation despite the same antigen are unclear. Possible explanations include different amounts of antigen, chronicity of the immune response, and differences in the immunoregulatory responses as well as genetic factors. Although categorization according to vessel size, organ system involvement, and the presence or absence of granulomata or eosinophils is useful, the three disease entities (classic PAN, allergic angiitis and granulomatosis, and the overlap syndrome) in this group have in common the fact that they are all *systemic necrotizing vasculitides*. The potential of devastating, life-threatening disease is present in all three. The failure to conform precisely to a well-defined clinical entity should not delay appropriate diagnostic and therapeutic measures. In this regard, clinical and therapeutic considerations in the overlap syndrome are similar to those described for classic PAN and allergic necrotizing vasculitis.

CHAPTER 5

HYPERSENSITIVITY VASCULITIS

INTRODUCTION

The hypersensitivity vasculitides, a heterogeneous group of clinical syndromes that have in common inflammation of small blood vessels, will be reviewed in three major sections. The first section will give a general overview of hypersensitivity vasculitis. The second will cover distinct clinical syndromes within the hypersensitivity vasculitis group, such as serum sickness, drug reactions, and Henoch-Schönlein purpura. The causative agents of these clinical syndromes are exogenous antigens such as drugs, foreign proteins, food, or microbes. Finally, the third section will review diseases in which hypersensitivity vasculitis may be part of a systemic illness (connective tissue disorders, selected malignancies, and certain autoimmune diseases). The hypersensitivity vasculitis in these diseases is characterized by an immune response to endogenous antigens such as autologous immunoglobulins, DNA, and, possibly, tumor antigens.

HYPERSENSITIVITY VASCULITIS

Definition.   Hypersensitivity vasculitis, which includes a heterogeneous group of clinical syndromes, is characterized by inflammation of small vessels such as arterioles, capillaries, and venules.[1] The vessel most commonly affected is the venule, producing a venulitis; less commonly, arterioles and capillaries are the primary sites of involvement. In comparison, classic polyarteritis nodosa (PAN) involves small- and intermediate-sized muscular arteries. Hypersensitivity vasculitis may affect any organ system, but skin involvement

50

dominates the clinical picture. With rare exceptions, this group of vasculitic diseases does not progress to life-threatening complications.

The term "hypersensitivity vasculitis" derives from the observation that in many patients with this syndrome the aberrant inflammatory response can be traced to a precipitating antigen such as a drug, foreign protein, or microbe.[214] In reality, a "hypersensitivity mechanism" may be involved in a number of vasculitic processes; however, "hypersensitivity vasculitis" continues to denote the clinical syndromes discussed in this chapter. Synonyms for this group of diseases include allergic vasculitis and leukocytoclastic vasculitis as well as several others.

Historical perspective. The historical aspects of the concept of hypersensitivity vasculitis have been reviewed in detail by Zeek,[4] who established the hypersensitivity vasculitis group as a separate entity.[5] Two major events were important in the identification of this group of vasculitides: (1) the study of two experimental models of vasculitis, namely, the Arthus reaction and the animal models of serum sickness, which established that exogenous antigens could produce vascular lesions similar to those seen in hypersensitivity vasculitis; and (2) the use of heterologous proteins and drugs (particularly horse serum and sulfonamides) that were associated with vasculitis, which was reflected predominantly in cutaneous vasculitic lesions in certain patients (reviewed in Chapter 2).

Incidence and prevalence. As with the larger vessel vasculitides, it is difficult to establish both an incidence and a prevalence for the hypersensitivity vasculitides. As a group, however, they are clearly more common than the systemic necrotizing vasculitis of the PAN group. The sex incidence varies with different reports, but in two large series[215, 216] a slight female predominance was noted. Frequently, association with a precipitating event, such as drug ingestion or infection, is noted. However, a precipitating antigen cannot be identified in all cases, and in some series, not even in the majority of cases.

Pathophysiology. Hypersensitivity vasculitis is an immunologic response to antigenic material. Evidence for this mechanism includes (1) well-studied animal models, (2) demonstration of antigenic material associated with immunoreactive proteins (i.e., immunoglobulins and complement) in skin biopsies of vasculitic lesions, and (3) temporal association between the exposure to a potentially antigenic material and the development of vasculitic lesions.

The mechanism for immune complex–mediated vasculitis in the animal model has been reviewed in Chapter 2. Briefly, the characteristics include (1) circulating immune complexes greater than 19S in size, (2) vasodilatation produced by one of several mechanisms, (3) deposition of immune complexes in the vessel wall with activation of

complement, and (4) influx of polymorphonuclear (PMN) leukocytes.[17] In the animal models, deposition of immune complexes can be
seen in small vessels, similar to the pattern seen in hypersensitivity
vasculitis, as well as in muscular arteries, similar to the pattern seen in
classic PAN. The reasons for deposition of immune complexes in
different-sized vessels are unclear at present.

Attempts have been made to demonstrate antigenic material in
human vascular lesions. Antigenic material from infectious agents,
such as hepatitis B surface antigen[65] and streptococcal, staphylococcal,
and mycobacterial organisms,[68, 69] has been demonstrated in human
vasculitic skin lesions. In addition, immune complexes and immunoglobulins (including IgG, IgA, and IgM) as well as complement
components can be demonstrated in the majority of vasculitic skin
lesions by immunofluorescent techniques[217-219] and electron microscopy.[217] Immunoglobulin and complement can be demonstrated in
vessel walls in biopsies of normal skin in patients with an active
cutaneous vasculitis,[217, 218] suggesting that the deposition of these
immunoreactive agents predates the vascular lesion. Of interest is
the fact that injection of histamine into an area of normal skin of a
patient with active vasculitis in other areas of the skin can result in
the appearance of a vasculitic lesion at the site of injection which is
demonstrable by biopsy.[217] This finding suggests that an additional
event beyond deposition of immunoglobulin and complement is
required for the full clinical expression of cutaneous vasculitis.
Clearly, increased vascular permeability plays a role in this series of
events by predisposing to the deposition of immune complexes in the
walls of the small vessels.

Various agents have been postulated as etiologic factors in hypersensitivity vasculitis.[214, 215, 220-223] A partial list would include (1)
infectious agents (*Streptococcus, Staphylococcus,* hepatitis B, influenza virus, cytomegalovirus, malaria, and mycobacterial organisms); (2) foreign proteins (animal serum and hyposensitization antigens); (3) chemicals (insecticides, herbicides, and petroleum
products); and (4) drugs (aspirin, phenacetin, phenothiazines, penicillin, sulfonamides, iodides, griseofulvin, tetracyclines, erythromy-
cin, propylthiouracil, and quinidine). Frequently, these agents are
implicated by association; for instance, a patient may receive a drug
and subsequently develop a cutaneous vasculitic eruption within a
time frame consistent with an immune-mediated response.

Rarely has an alternative mechanism been suggested for vasculitic skin lesions. Cold-induced urticaria with a leukocytoclastic pattern
on biopsy has been reported,[216] and has been studied in one patient in
detail.[224] Clinically, the patient had flexion contractures of the fingers
and toes, dermographism, and depressed serum complement as well
as the cold-induced urticaria. Sequential biopsies of the cold-induced
lesions demonstrated massive degranulation of mast cells initially,

followed by sequential infiltration by neutrophilic, eosinophilic, and basophilic PMN leukocytes. The authors postulated a combination of pathologic processes involving mast cells and the classic complement system. Again, a physical stress, such as cold, may rarely lead to cutaneous vasculitis with a histologic appearance of hypersensitivity vasculitis.

Clinical considerations.   Hypersensitivity vasculitis is seen at all ages. The mean age in one series[216] was 47 years with a range of from 3 to 68 years. In another series[215] the majority of patients were between the ages of 30 and 60 years. Fever is seen in the minority of cases, being present in 20 per cent of patients.[215] Except as noted, the following summary of clinical manifestations reflects the experience of Winkelmann and Ditto[215] and Cream,[216] who altogether reported on a total of 73 patients.

CUTANEOUS DISEASE.   The cutaneous manifestations of hypersensitivity vasculitis are presented in Table 5–1. The classic lesion is the so-called palpable purpura seen in Figure 5–1, and evidence for intracutaneous bleeding is found in almost all cases. Papular and

TABLE 5–1.   MANIFESTATIONS OF CUTANEOUS DISEASE IN HYPERSENSITIVITY VASCULITIS*

MANIFESTATIONS	PERCENTAGE OF INVOLVEMENT	NUMBER OF OBSERVATIONS†
Classification of Lesions		
Hemorrhage into skin/purpura	99	73
Papule/petechiae	37	38
Necrotic ulceration	29	73
Vesicles/bullae	21	73
Urticaria	9	35
Erythema multiforme	9	35
Nodule	8	38
Livedo reticularis	3	73
Distribution of Lesions		
Feet and ankles	100	38
Face	16	38
Mucosal membranes	16	38
Ear	11	38
Conjunctivae	5	38
Symptomatic Complaints		
Dependent edema	47	38
Asymptomatic	32	38
Burning or stinging	24	38
Pain	13	38

*Data in this table are summarized from references 215 and 216, which review a total of 73 patients.

†Number of patients for whom a given observation was evaluated.

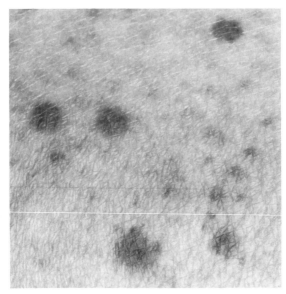

Figure 5–1. Characteristic pattern of "palpable purpura" seen on the lower extremity of a patient with chronic recurrent hypersensitivity vasculitis. Purpuric lesions 2 to 5 mm in diameter are seen.

petechial as well as ulcerative lesions can also be seen. Less common lesions include vesicles, bullae, urticaria, erythema multiforme, nodules, and livedo reticularis. A pattern of an urticarial papule surrounded by petechial lesions was noted in another series.[215]

The lesions tend to appear in recurrent crops varying in number from 1 to more than 100. The size varies from several millimeters to several centimeters. The lesion may go through an evolutionary cycle, beginning as a petechia or papule, progressing to a hemorrhagic vesicular or bullous stage, and ending as a nodular or plaque-like lesion. In some cases, progression to ulceration follows the plaque stage. After recurrent episodes, macular pigmentation may be seen. Each crop of lesions may take from several weeks to over 1 month to fully resolve.

The lesions tend to have a symmetric distribution and are most frequently found in dependent areas, particularly the distal lower extremities. Involvement of the thighs and buttocks is common. Lesions in the upper extremities may also be noted, particularly around the wrist. Less frequently, lesions on the face, mucosal membranes, ears, and conjunctivae can be seen.

The skin lesions are associated with pain or a burning sensation in approximately 40 per cent of patients. Approximately one third of patients note no symptoms related to the cutaneous lesions. Dependent edema, which was frequently associated with discomfort or frank pain, is described in approximately one half the patients in one series.[215]

A clinical syndrome characterized by urticarial lesions with a biopsy pattern of venulitis has been reviewed in detail.[225-227] This clinical syndrome is remarkable for rapid resolution of lesions (1 to 3 days), female preponderance, frequent joint symptoms (particularly arthralgias), abdominal pain, and rare renal involvement. The finding of vasculitis on skin biopsies from patients with chronic recurrent urticaria is not unusual and was present in one half the patients in one series.[228, 229]

It is difficult to reliably define the frequency of systemic involvement in patients with true hypersensitivity vasculitis. In the large clinical series of patients with cutaneous vasculitis by Winkelmann and Ditto[215] and Cream,[216] patients with systemic vasculitic syndromes such as classic PAN and allergic angiitis and granulomatosis, as well as patients with other systemic illnesses such as Sjögren's syndrome, are included in the discussion. Information on patients with cutaneous vasculitis in whom large vessel vasculitis and other systemic illnesses have been carefully excluded is not currently available; consequently, the frequency of organ system involvement discussed in the following paragraphs reflects the experience in this heterogeneous group of patients with vasculitis.[215, 216] In our experience, systemic involvement in patients with the true hypersensitivity vasculitis syndrome is significantly less frequent than that currently reported in the medical literature. Again, it is important to emphasize that when systemic involvement is present in patients with true hypersensitivity vasculitis, clinically significant organ system dysfunction is unusual.

JOINT. Arthritis or arthralgia is seen in approximately 40 per cent of patients. One or several joints may be involved, with knees, ankles, wrists, and elbows the most commonly affected sites. Progression to chronic, deforming arthritis is not seen.

KIDNEY. Renal involvement is present in 37 per cent of cases, with asymptomatic hematuria being the most common presentation. Compromise of renal function is seen in approximately 10 per cent of patients. In one series,[215] three of the four deaths related to active disease were caused by renal failure. Of note, two of these four patients had vascular lesions of the muscular arteries in the kidneys or bowel, thus establishing a diagnosis of PAN and putting these patients in the category of systemic vasculitis and not typical hypersensitivity vasculitis.

LUNG. Pulmonary abnormalities may be seen in 19 per cent of cases with nonspecific patterns of infiltrates or pleural effusions or both seen on chest radiographs. The significance of the radiographic findings with regard to disease activity is unclear. Pulmonary vasculitis was not seen in the four cases evaluated at autopsy, including the one case with a pulmonary infiltrate diagnosed prior to death.[215]

GASTROINTESTINAL TRACT. Involvement of the bowel is present in 15 per cent of cases, with evidence of bleeding (melena or hematemesis) being the most common presentation. No life-threatening surgical emergencies from bowel involvement were noted.

NERVOUS SYSTEM. The most common lesions, a peripheral neuropathy, are seen in 12 per cent of cases. Cerebrovascular accidents are reported in 5 per cent of cases in one series,[215] although it is unclear if this finding is directly related to the hypersensitivity vasculitis.

HEART. Rarely, pericarditis is present. Myocarditis, if it exists in association with hypersensitivity vasculitis, is exceedingly rare.

Laboratory. No specific laboratory test is diagnostic of hypersensitivity vasculitis. In general, there is a mild leukocytosis and elevated erythrocyte sedimentation rate (ESR). Eosinophilia may be seen but is not characteristic. Cryoglobulins and rheumatoid factor are present in a variable number of cases. Serum complement levels may be normal or depressed, but no pattern is diagnostic.

Pathology. The most common histologic pattern is a PMN leukocyte infiltrate of postcapillary venules with leukocytoclasis (presence of nuclear debris), fibrinoid necrosis, endothelial swelling, and extravasation of erythrocytes into the perivascular areas (Fig. 5–2).[215, 220] The damaged vessels in hypersensitivity vasculitis are usually at the same stage of involvement, suggesting a "burst" of immune complex deposition. In comparison, the vasculitic lesions in PAN are usually in all stages of development.

Two distinct cellular patterns in cutaneous vasculitis have been proposed.[73] The first is a pattern of predominantly neutrophilic infiltration associated with hypocomplementemia believed to be due to immune complex deposition. The second is a pattern of predominantly lymphocytic infiltration with normal complement, which is thought to be due to delayed hypersensitivity or cellular immune mechanisms. Other observers feel that the neutrophilic versus mononuclear infiltrates in small vessel vasculitis represent a continuous evolution from acute to chronic vasculitis and are not indicative of different mechanisms.[219, 230]

Although changes of small vessel angiitis are most commonly appreciated in the skin, this vasculitic process can potentially affect any organ system, usually to a much lesser extent. Characteristic clinicopathologic patterns related to different organs help to subdivide syndromes within hypersensitivity vasculitis. It is important to emphasize that the microinfarcts that characterize the hypersensitivity vasculitides do not generally cause major organ system dysfunction such as is usually seen in the systemic necrotizing vasculitides.

Diagnosis and differential diagnosis. The diagnosis of hypersensitivity vasculitis is established by finding small vessel involvement, usually with a leukocytoclastic pattern as described. The skin is the most common and readily biopsied site, although biopsies of symptomatic muscle groups may have a significant yield. As men-

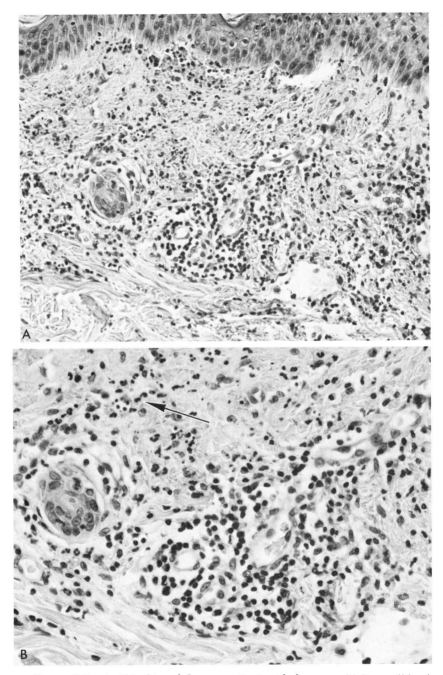

Figure 5–2. A, Skin biopsy from a patient with hypersensitivity angiitis. A venulitis with a mixed cellular infiltrate is seen. Hematoxylin and eosin stain (original magnification ×80). B, A more detailed view of the biopsy seen in A. Note that a mononuclear cell infiltrate around a venule is marked in one area of biopsy, while polymorphonuclear leukocytes with early leukocytoclasis (presence of nuclear debris) is seen in an adjacent area (arrow). Hematoxylin and eosin stain (original magnification ×330).

tioned earlier, any organ system may be involved and appropriate biopsies can confirm this involvement. Biopsies of affected kidneys usually show small vessel involvement or glomerulitis or both, with fibrinoid necrosis of the capillary loop.

It is very important to remember that a pattern of hypersensitivity vasculitis on skin biopsy may be associated with underlying systemic diseases; therefore, any patient with this skin lesion should have a complete evaluation. Diseases such as classic PAN, allergic angiitis and granulomatosis, overlap vasculitis syndrome,[1] systemic lupus erythematosus (SLE), Sjögren's syndrome, rheumatoid arthritis, and other collagen vascular diseases can be associated with cutaneous small vessel vasculitis and should be included in the differential diagnosis of patients with a hypersensitivity vasculitis on skin biopsy. Thus, the syndrome of "hypersensitivity vasculitis" is one in which the skin is predominantly involved. However, a number of systemic vasculitides can have skin involvement that is histopathologically indistinguishable from the skin involvement of hypersensitivity vasculitis.

Treatment and prognosis.   Since the hypersensitivity vasculitides comprise a somewhat heterogeneous group of disorders, the prognosis and treatment of each of these will vary according to the subcategory in question. Removal of the offending antigen, such as cessation of a suspect drug or treatment of an underlying infection, is adequate if such an agent can be identified. Because certain categories of hypersensitivity vasculitis manifest a tendency toward spontaneous resolution in some cases, there are few data to indicate that any mode of therapy consistently alters the course of these diseases.[220] Chronic, recurrent cases of cutaneous vasculitis may be refractory to a wide range of therapeutic agents. Even aggressive immunosuppressive therapy with corticosteroids and cytotoxic agents may not produce clinical remission. In patients with significant systemic involvement, particularly renal disease, corticosteroid therapy is recommended. Generally, prednisone given orally, 40 to 60 mg per day with tapering according to disease activity, is attempted. In patients with disease refractory to steroid therapy or progressive dysfunction of a vital organ system (i.e., declining renal function), immunosuppressive agents have been tried. The efficacy of these agents in hypersensitivity vasculitis is not well established.

In general, the prognosis in hypersensitivity vasculitis is good with or without therapy. With the exception of the few patients who progress to renal failure, hypersensitivity vasculitis is generally not a life-threatening disease.

SUBGROUPS OF HYPERSENSITIVITY VASCULITIS

Several subgroups of hypersensitivity vasculitis have distinctive clinicopathologic characteristics and thus have historically been referred to as separate syndromes. In this section, serum sickness, Henoch-Schönlein purpura, and "vasculitis with mixed cryoglobulinemia with an established exogenous antigen" will be covered in more detail. Remember that these diseases are part of a spectrum of true hypersensitivity vasculitides and are characterized by a response to an exogenous antigen.

SERUM SICKNESS AND "SERUM SICKNESS–LIKE" REACTIONS

Definition. Serum sickness is a clinical syndrome that results from injection of foreign or heterologous serum or serum proteins into an individual. The clinicopathologic presentation of serum sickness in man closely parallels the animal models.[16, 17] Clinical serum sickness is rarely seen today, reflecting the infrequent use of heterologous serum as a therapeutic agent in man. A clinical syndrome similar, if not identical, to classic serum sickness is seen rarely after the administration of non–protein-containing drugs. Penicillin[231] and sulfapyridine[232] have been implicated in this syndrome, which is often referred to as a serum sickness–like reaction. Rarely, other non–protein-containing drugs, including sulfonamides, streptomycin, thiouracils, and hydantoin compounds,[221] may also be involved.

Incidence and prevalence. Historically, heterologous serum was extensively used to treat pneumococcal pneumonia and diphtheria, and for prophylaxis following exposure to tetanus. Current uses of heterologous serum are quite limited and include prophylaxis for botulism, gas gangrene, rabies, and snakebite. Heterologous antilymphocyte serum for organ transplant rejection has been used extensively and is another potential source of serum sickness. However, the incidence of full-blown serum sickness in this setting is relatively infrequent, perhaps owing to the immunosuppressed status of the patient population. In essence, classic serum sickness is a rare disease today.

On the other hand, the frequency of serum sickness–like reactions to non–protein-containing drugs is difficult to establish. The frequency of drug reactions in hospitalized patients is 15 per cent,[221] suggesting that serum sickness–like reactions may not be quite so rare.

Pathophysiology. Immune complex deposition is undoubtedly responsible for the widespread vasculitic lesions seen in serum sickness.[233] In general, the frequency and severity of the serum sickness reaction are directly related to the volume of foreign protein injected.[234] Although less well established, the presumptive mechanism for serum sickness–like reactions is mediation by immune complexes. The urticarial component of the cutaneous manifestations of serum sickness may be mediated by IgE with or without immune complex deposition.

Clinical manifestations. The classic clinical manifestations of

serum sickness consist of fever, urticaria, arthralgias, and lymphadenopathy. A small percentage of patients may develop a clinical picture
of disseminated vasculitis, glomerulonephritis, and peripheral neuritis. The onset of symptoms following exposure to heterologous serum
varies with individuals. Generally, patients experience a pruritic
erythematous swelling at the injection site 1 to 3 days before the more
generalized symptoms are apparent. The full clinical syndrome occurs
7 to 10 days following primary exposure to the antigen, although
delays of 2 to 3 weeks have been noted. Accelerated reactions with a
systemic response in 1 to 4 days may be seen in patients with histories
of prior exposure. The finding of low-titer IgG antibody against
heterologous serum proteins increases the patient's risk of developing
serum sickness, including an accelerated reaction.[235] Clinical improvement in the majority of cases starts in 2 to 4 days, with complete
resolution in 1 to 2 weeks.

Functional impairment of major organ systems is rare. Proteinuria
may be found in some cases, but clinically significant renal dysfunction is rare. However, following exposure to large doses of equine
serum, fatal glomerulonephritis has been reported.[236] Rare complications include carditis, coronary arteritis, peripheral neuropathy (including brachial neuritis), encephalitis, and a clinical picture of
ascending paralysis (reviewed in reference 235).

Laboratory considerations.   A mild leukocytosis and an elevated
ESR are common. Leukopenia is less frequently seen, and eosinophilia may or may not be present. Evidence for an exuberant immunologic
response in the form of hypergammaglobulinemia, plasmacytosis, and
circulating light chains has been demonstrated.[237] IgG antibodies
against heterologous serum proteins can be demonstrated by hemag-
glutination in some cases.[235] Joint fluid analysis of involved joints is
nondiagnostic but tends to have an inflammatory pattern.

Diagnosis and differential diagnosis.   The diagnosis of serum
sickness is suggested when the characteristic clinical syndrome is
seen following exposure to a foreign protein or drug. Demonstrating
IgG antibodies to a suspect antigen helps to confirm the diagnosis.
The clinical manifestations of serum sickness, particularly mild reactions, could be confused with a wide variety of infectious or inflammatory diseases.

Treatment and prognosis.   The majority of serum sickness and
serum sickness–like reactions resolve spontaneously in from several
days to 2 weeks after removal of the offending antigen. Antihistamines
may provide symptomatic relief from pruritus, and aspirin in analgesic
doses usually controls most joint-related symptoms. A brief course of
corticosteroids, such as prednisone given orally 40 to 60 mg per day
with a rapid taper, has been employed to suppress symptoms in the
more severe cases.

The prognosis in serum sickness is excellent, with spontaneous
resolution in nearly all cases. Fatal reactions are exceedingly rare now

that large doses, such as 200 ml of serum, are no longer given. A history of serum sickness or a serum sickness–like reaction to a given drug is a strong contraindication to re-exposure.

HENOCH-SCHÖNLEIN PURPURA

Definition. Henoch-Schönlein purpura is a distinctive subgroup of the hypersensitivity vasculitides and is characterized by the clinicopathologic complex of nonthrombocytopenic purpura, skin lesions, joint involvement, colicky abdominal pain with gastrointestinal hemorrhage, and renal disease.[1, 238] This syndrome has been referred to by various names, including Schönlein's purpura, Henoch's purpura, Osler's syndrome, anaphylactoid purpura, allergic purpura, purpura rheumatica, nonthrombocytopenic purpura, acute vascular purpura, vascular anaphylactoid purpura, primary purpura, and urticarial purpura (reviewed in reference 239). Within the spectrum of hypersensitivity vasculitides, Henoch-Schönlein purpura is a systemic small vessel vasculitis.

Historical perspective. The original clinical descriptions were reported by Heberden[240] and Willan.[241] Schönlein[242] recognized a distinct syndrome characterized by rash and joint symptoms. Henoch[243] described the abdominal symptoms and gastrointestinal blood loss and in a subsequent report[244] described the renal component of the syndrome. Osler[245] suggested a clinical similarity between Henoch-Schönlein purpura and serum sickness. Glanzmann[246] recognized that infection and sensitization may be important in this syndrome and Gairdner[247] has reviewed the historical evolution of Henoch-Schönlein purpura in detail.

Incidence and prevalence. Henoch-Schönlein purpura is not a rare disorder. Several authors have recently published large series of articles on patients with this disease.[248–250] In one series,[251] Henoch-Schönlein purpura accounted for between 5 and 24 admissions per year at a pediatric hospital. Most patients range in age from 4 to 7 years,[248, 251] but the disease is seen in infants as well as adults.[249] The clinical manifestations do vary somewhat with age. In patients less than 2 years old, localized edema (particularly around the face and scalp) is common, while intussusception and renal failure are exceedingly rare. In children 4 to 5 years old, the risk of intussusception is greatest. In adults, joint symptoms are prominent and the risk of functional renal impairment appears to be greater.[249] The disease is more common in males, with a ratio of 1.5 to 1 (Table 5–2), and a seasonal variation with a peak incidence in spring has been noted.[251]

Pathophysiology. The presumptive mechanism for Henoch-Schönlein purpura involves immune complex deposition. Multiple possible antigens have been suggested. Approximately two thirds of

TABLE 5-2. CLINICAL PARAMETERS FOR PEDIATRIC PATIENTS WITH HENOCH-SCHÖNLEIN PURPURA°

CLINICAL PARAMETERS	RESULTS	NUMBER OF OBSERVATIONS†
General Considerations		
Male to female ratio	1.5 to 1	218
	Per cent	
Fever	75	131
Hypertension	13	206
Organ System Involvement		
Skin	100	218
Purpura	100	218
Ulceration	4	75
Joints	71	218
Gastrointestinal tract	68	218
Pain	57	64
Nausea, vomiting	50	12
Occult blood	42	206
Hematemesis/melena	35	218
Major bleed	5	131
Intussusception	3	131
Kidney		
Hematuria	45	218
Microscopic	45	218
Macroscopic	26	218
Proteinuria	35	218
Functional impairment	9	131
Localized edema	32	206

°This table summarizes the experience with 218 patients reported in references 247, 248, and 251.

†Number of patients for whom a given observation was evaluated

patients have symptoms of an upper respiratory tract infection prior to onset of their disease,[248, 251] suggesting that infectious agents may be important. Evidence of a streptococcal infection is present in 20 per cent of patients.[249, 251] Prior drug therapy, particularly with penicillin, tetracycline, sulfonamides, aspirin, or thiazides, is frequently noted.[251, 252] Various foods have been implicated as a source of antigen, including milk, eggs, wheat, rice, fish, nuts, beans, and others.[253-256] Henoch-Schönlein purpura has also been associated with insect bites,[257] smallpox vaccination,[258, 259] influenza vaccination,[260] and exposure to cold.[261, 262]

Elevated levels of circulating IgA were initially noted in a substantial number of patients within 3 months of onset of the disease.[90] Subsequently, IgA as well as C3 was demonstrated in blood vessels from both involved and adjacent normal skin.[263, 264] Additional observations in this disease include increased numbers of IgA-bearing lymphocytes in the peripheral circulation and IgA-containing circulating immune complexes.[103, 265] These observations strongly suggest an IgA immune complex–mediated disease.

Deposition of IgA has been demonstrated in the renal biopsy of patients with Henoch-Schönlein purpura.[263, 266] The IgA is generally localized in the renal mesangium.[263] Although IgA immune complexes may be important in mediation of the renal disease, the full spectrum of pathophysiologic mechanisms may be quite complex. In one series, only those patients with both circulating IgA and IgG immune complexes developed the nephritic component of the disease.[103] Moreover, other diseases, such as lupus nephritis and Buerger's disease,[266, 267] are associated with renal IgA deposition. Mechanisms other than immune complex deposition could conceivably be involved; for example, primary deposition of antigen in the mesangium followed by an antibody response,[268] as well as antibody directed against mesangial determinants,[269] has been described.

IgA antibody has several immunoreactive properties that could be significant in the pathophysiology of Henoch-Schönlein purpura. Specifically, IgA can bind to PMN leukocytes,[270] suppress PMN chemotaxis,[271] and activate the complement system by the alternate pathway.[272] Several clinicopathologic observations in Henoch-Schönlein purpura have suggested a role for activation of complement by the alternate pathway. In cutaneous vessels or renal mesangium or both, C3 and properdin factor B can be demonstrated in the absence of the early components of the classic complement pathway, namely, C1 and C4.[264, 267] Moreover, Henoch-Schönlein purpura has been described in patients with congenital absence of C2.[273, 274] Since chemotactic influx of PMN leukocytes in vessel walls is believed to require C3, activation of the complement system by the alternate pathway plays an important role in the mediation of this disease. The association between an upper respiratory tract infection and the apparent importance of IgA in the mediation of Henoch-Schönlein purpura is of interest. It is possible that an abnormal local immune response of IgA to an infectious agent in the respiratory tract may produce IgA immune complex–mediated disease. In a similar fashion, food may provide an antigenic stimulus for an abnormal immune response of IgA in the gastrointestinal tract, producing IgA immune complex–mediated disease.

Clinical considerations. Clinical parameters for pediatric and adult patients with Henoch-Schönlein purpura are summarized in Tables 5–2 and 5–3, respectively. In pediatric patients, presenting symptoms related to the skin, gut, and joints are present in 50 per cent of cases.[247] In the adult group, presenting symptoms related to the skin are seen in over 70 per cent of patients, while initial complaints related to the gut or the joints are noted in less than 20 per cent of cases.[252]

SKIN. Involvement of the skin is noted at some point in almost

TABLE 5–3.   CLINICAL PARAMETERS FOR ADULTS WITH
HENOCH-SCHÖNLEIN PURPURA*

CLINICAL PARAMETERS	RESULTS	NUMBER OF OBSERVATIONS†
General Considerations		
Age (mean)	44.7	91
	Per cent	
Fever	50	14
Hypertension	22	14
Organ System Involvement		
Skin	100	91
Purpura	100	91
Maculopapular lesions	62	77
Ulceration	16	77
Joints	73	78
Kidney	61	64
Gastrointestinal tract	53	78
Pain	41	64
Occult blood	21	78
Hematemesis/melena	19	64
Diarrhea	19	64
Nausea/vomiting	16	64
Lung	6	64

*This table summarizes the experience with 91 patients reported in references 249 and 252.
†Number of patients for whom a given observation was evaluated

all cases and tends to have a symmetric distribution. The major sites are the extremities (Table 5–4), with greater involvement seen distally on the extensor surfaces; the lower extremities are affected more frequently. Lesions around the buttocks are seen in approximately 50 per cent of cases, but involvement of the trunk or mucosal membranes is less frequent. The cutaneous lesions of Henoch-Schönlein purpura have been described in detail.[247] Initially, there is a small urticarial lesion on the extensor surface which may be pruritic; it evolves within hours to a pink maculopapular spot. The lesion then darkens and may

TABLE 5–4.   DISTRIBUTION OF CUTANEOUS LESIONS IN
HENOCH-SCHÖNLEIN PURPURA*

SITE	PERCENTAGE OF INVOLVEMENT	NUMBER OF OBSERVATIONS†
Leg	95	152
Arm	58	77
Buttock	45	152
Trunk	12	77
Mucosa	Rare	–

*Data summarized are taken from references 248 and 249.
†Number of patients for which a given observation was evaluated

become raised, and by the following day there is a maculopapular lesion from 0.5 to 2 cm in size, which may or may not progress to a confluent patch. Resolution requires approximately 2 weeks, during which time the purpural lesion turns to a brown-colored macule and then finally heals without scarring.

EXTREMITIES. Symptoms related to the joints are seen in the majority of cases, with involvement of knees, ankles, wrists, and elbows in descending order of frequency. One or several joints may be affected, and a migratory pattern with sequential involvement of different joints has been noted. In general, the joint involvement is mild in the younger patients and more extensive in adult patients.[249] Bleeding into the calf muscle has been noted in several series.[248, 251]

ABDOMEN. Clinical involvement of the gastrointestinal tract is seen in approximately 70 per cent of pediatric patients and 50 per cent of adult patients (Table 5–3). The most common finding is pain, which tends to have a colicky quality, but nausea, vomiting, and blood loss are also quite frequent. Major gastrointestinal tract hemorrhage requiring multiple transfusions may be seen in 5 per cent of cases. Symptoms related to the abdomen may precede skin involvement in 10 to 15 per cent.[248, 275] In the majority of patients the pain is probably related to small vessel vasculitis with hemorrhage into the bowel wall. Rarely, pancreatitis may complicate a case of Henoch-Schönlein purpura.[276, 277] Loss of protein through the bowel has also been described in adult patients.[247]

Rare complications, such as nonreducible intussusception or bowel perforation, will require surgical intervention.[278-280] The decision between laparotomy and conservative management is a difficult one. The most common form of intussusception is ileoileal; however, ileocolic and ileocecal patterns have also been reported.[279] The mean age for patients with this complication is approximately 6 years, but it can also be seen in young adults.[278] Intussusception with Henoch-Schönlein purpura appears to be rare in children less than 3 years of age and in older adults.[278, 281] Clinically, the diagnosis of intussusception is suggested in a patient with a worsening clinical course, an unchanging abdominal mass, bright red blood per rectum, and a clinical pattern of complete bowel obstruction.[278] Surgical intervention for Henoch-Schönlein purpura–related intussusception is associated with a mortality rate of 13 per cent, while the nonoperative mortality rate is 55 per cent. Bowel perforation is also associated with a high mortality rate.[278]

KIDNEY. Renal involvement is usually characterized by mild hematuria and is generally not part of the presenting clinical picture. It usually resolves spontaneously without therapy. Rarely, a progressive glomerulonephritis will develop. Renal failure is the most common cause of death in the rare patient who dies of Henoch-Schönlein purpura.[248, 249, 252]

EDEMA. Edema may be present in a third of the cases. In infants there tend to be localized patches of swelling around the scalp, face, neck, hands, scrotum, or feet.[248] In adults, generalized dependent edema may be present.[249]

Rarely, other major organ systems may be involved. In adults, pulmonary involvement is present in 6 per cent of patients, with hemoptysis and pleuritic complaints being recorded.[249] Rarely, carditis is described,[282] but in the presence of an elevated anti–streptolysin O titer, rheumatic heart disease may explain this finding. Central nervous system involvement has also been reported with vasculitis,[247] subarachnoid bleeding, and intracerebral hemorrhage,[283] although these complications are quite rare.

Laboratory considerations. Routine laboratory studies generally show a mild leukocytosis, a normal platelet count, and, occasionally, eosinophilia. The ESR is elevated in approximately one third of patients.[248, 252] Microscopic hematuria, proteinuria, and red cell casts in the urine can be found in the majority of patients. Renal function abnormalities are less frequent. Elevated immunoglobulins, particularly IgA, may be seen in one half the cases.[90]

Roentgenographic studies of the bowel may be helpful in diagnosing an intussusception. Filling defects, loss of mucosal pattern, and narrowing of bowel lumen may also be observed.[284] Generally, there is complete resolution of the radiographic abnormalities, but, rarely, stricture with fibrosis and obstruction has been reported.[285]

Pathology. The histopathology of this disease is characterized by a diffuse leukocytoclastic vasculitis involving small vessels of essentially all organ systems but predominantly the skin, joints, gastrointestinal tract, and kidneys. Hemorrhage with purpuric lesions is characteristic. In the bowel, hemorrhage may be seen in the submucosal or the subserosal areas together with multiple ulcers along the bowel mucosa.[286] Intussusception probably results from submucosal hemorrhage or fluid extravasation with subsequent protrusion in the gut lumen. Renal histopathology usually consists of focal or diffuse glomerulonephritis.

Diagnosis and differential diagnosis. The combination of the characteristic skin lesions, a normal platelet count, and joint and gastrointestinal symptoms with or without renal involvement should suggest the diagnosis of Henoch-Schönlein purpura. A skin biopsy will establish the vasculitic nature of the process, and immunofluorescent studies showing IgA deposition in vessel walls will further support the diagnosis. The differential diagnosis for a patient presenting with rash, abdominal pain, and joint symptoms would include inflammatory bowel disease, *Yersinia* enterocolitis, meningococcemia, Rocky Mountain spotted fever, rheumatic fever, hepatitis B infection, and mononucleosis as well as other diseases.[287] The differential diagnosis in those cases in which the abdominal symptoms predominate includes all diseases that can produce an acute abdomen.

Treatment and prognosis. Because the disease usually resolves spontaneously after one to several recurrent episodes, the prognosis even in an untreated patient is excellent. Therapy consists of supportive care and symptomatic relief. If an infectious agent is identified, an appropriate drug should be started. Any particular food implicated as a source of antigen should be eliminated from the diet. Corticosteroid therapy may be effective in reducing local edema and in suppressing gastrointestinal and joint symptoms.[248, 288] Aspirin is ineffective in suppressing symptoms and may increase the risk of bleeding. Bed rest has also been suggested, particularly if renal failure is present.[255] There is no good evidence to suggest that corticosteroids affect the outcome in patients with altered renal function,[289] and immunosuppressive therapy also seems to produce a variable response.[290, 291] However, in the rare case in which there is progressive deterioration in renal function despite corticosteroid therapy, a trial of cytotoxic therapy may be warranted.

"Vasculitis with Mixed Cryoglobulinemia"

Definition. The diseases in this group were originally referred to as essential mixed cryoglobulinemias.[104, 292, 293] However, with the demonstration of exogenous antigens (namely, hepatitis B antigen[66] and coccidioidin antigen[106] in the cryoprecipitate of certain patients with this disease), the descriptive term "essential" is no longer appropriate for all patients with mixed cryoglobulinemia and vasculitis. "Vasculitis with mixed cryoglobulinemia" is the preferred term to describe this subgroup of patients within the spectrum of hypersensitivity vasculitis in whom the antigen has been identified. However, it is important to emphasize that the patients in whom antigenic material, such as hepatitis B antigen or coccidioidin antigen, can be identified in the cryoprecipitate represent only a fraction of the total number with vasculitis associated with mixed cryoglobulinemia. Strictly speaking, there is still a category of this disease that is essential.

Clinically, this disease presents with weakness, a purpural rash on the lower extremities, and symptoms related to joints with or without a glomerulonephritis. A cryoglobulin with a type II or "mixed" pattern[105, 294] can be isolated from the patient's serum. The type II pattern consists of polyclonal IgG and, generally, a monoclonal IgM with rheumatoid factor (anti-Fc) activity. Rarely, the monoclonal component will be an IgA or IgG. Attempts to define an exogenous antigen will be successful in only a fraction of cases, leaving a significant group of patients with no established external antigen. Vasculitis with mixed cryoglobulinemia is characterized by small vessel vasculitis of the skin and immune cryoprecipitable complexes with a type II or mixed pattern in the serum. The clinical presentation and the histologic appearance of the cutaneous vasculitis are similar for patients with or without an identified exogenous antigen.

Vasculitis with mixed cryoglobulinemia has only relatively recently been defined; therefore, its relationship to the group of hypersensitivity vasculitides as a whole has not been clearly established. Cryoglobulins may be present in patients with hypersensitivity vasculitis[216] and Henoch-Schönlein purpura.[252] The relationship to other syndromes associated with cryoglobulinemia, such as the "hypergammaglobulinemic purpura" described by Capra and colleagues,[295] will require additional studies.

Eventually, additional antigens will undoubtedly be defined. In this regard, Levo and colleagues[66] identified a virus-like particle on electron microscopic evaluation of a cryoglobulin which was negative for both hepatitis B antigen and antibody, suggesting another viral antigen. Epstein-Barr virus and cytomegalovirus infections as well as chronic infections (such as syphilis, lymphogranuloma venereum, and leprosy) can be associated with cryoglobulinemia. Evaluation of cryoprecipitates for these pathogens as well as others may be productive.

Pathophysiology.   There is strong evidence that this disease is mediated by immune complex deposition. Immunofluorescent studies in both renal and cutaneous biopsies of vasculitic lesions have demonstrated the presence of IgM, IgG, and C3.[104, 293] Serum complement levels may also be depressed, suggesting complement utilization.[296]

The composition of the mixed cryoglobulins deserves further comment. Levo et al.[66] demonstrated that the polyclonal IgG had specific activity against hepatitis by surface antigen. The monoclonal IgM antibody, in addition to the anti-Fc piece activity, also has specific anti–hepatitis B surface antigen activity. The significance of these observations with respect to the pathophysiology of this disease is unclear. In this regard, cryoglobulins composed of IgM and IgG, including IgM antibody with rheumatoid factor activity,[297] can be found in sera from significant numbers of normal individuals. This finding suggests that this pattern of antibody production is a physiologic host response. Regulating antibody production and increasing the size of immune complexes to facilitate clearance are two possible functions for antibodies with anti-Fc activity.[105]

The physiochemical parameters of cryoprecipitable immunoglobulins have been reviewed in detail.[105] Of particular interest is the fact that the rheumatoid factor activity may vary with temperature, showing increased activity at lower temperatures.[298] This property may, in part, be responsible for the localization of vasculitis to the extremities, where the temperature can be significantly lower than core temperatures.[105]

Clinical considerations.   Detailed clinical information on patients with vasculitis and mixed cryoglobulinemia is difficult to summarize because patients with a pattern of mixed cryoglobulinemia, whether or not they have vasculitis or another systemic illness, are frequently discussed as a single group. There appears to be a female predominance in patients with vasculitis and mixed cryoglobulinemia,[66, 104] and a mean age of 53 years is noted in one series.[66] A purpural skin rash involving the distal aspect of the lower extremities in the majority of cases is present in over 90 per cent of patients. The rash may be preceded by a burning or itching sensation[294] and may be precipitated by stress, standing, tight stockings, or exposure to cold. The lesions usually resolve in 1 to 2 weeks but may persist for several weeks. Symptoms related to joints are present in the majority of patients, but frank arthritis is less frequent. Renal involvement in the form of glomerulonephritis is seen in 50 per cent of patients and may progress to clinically significant functional renal impairment in some individuals.[66] Clinically significant liver disease is present in a minority of patients. Recently, the high incidence of lung involvement in this disease has been emphasized.[299] Most patients are asymptomatic, but hemoptysis, wheezing, and dyspnea can be noted occasionally. An interstitial pattern on chest film, a nonhomogeneous pattern on regional lung scan, and evidence of small airway disease from pulmonary function studies are characteristic. The clinical significance of these findings has not been determined. In addition, a peripheral neuropathy may be present.

Laboratory considerations. In general, laboratory tests are similar to those described for hypersensitivity vasculitis. There is generally a mild leukocytosis, usually an elevated erythrocyte sedimentation rate, and, less frequently, an eosinophilia. Demonstration of a type II cryoglobulinemia is required for the diagnosis, and an exogenous antigen may be identified in some patients. As noted previously, serum complement levels may be depressed.

Pathology. Biopsy of skin lesions shows a small vessel vasculitis characteristic of the hypersensitivity vasculitides. Similarly, renal biopsy abnormalities include a diffuse glomerulonephritis with cellular proliferation. Endomembranous deposits or acute vasculitis of small vessels or both may be seen in some cases.

Diagnosis and differential diagnosis. In a patient with a clinical picture of weakness, purpura, and joint symptoms, the diagnosis is established by demonstration of a type II cryoglobulin and a small vessel vasculitis on skin biopsy. The spectrum of cryoprecipitable proteins in human serum has been reviewed in detail.[105] Cryoglobulins must be distinguished from cryofibrinogen, cryoprecipitable light chains, and C-reactive protein-albumin complexes. Once the diagnosis of cryoglobulinemia is established, the distinction between type I (monoclonal), type II (mixed monoclonal-polyclonal), and type III (polyclonal) must be made. Finally, a variety of systemic diseases, including multiple myeloma, Waldenström's macroglobulinemia, Sjögren's syndrome, and SLE, may exhibit a type II pattern and must be excluded (reviewed in reference 105).

Treatment and prognosis. The long-term prognosis is good. The natural history of the disease includes recurrent attacks. Clinically significant hepatic disease, such as chronic active hepatitis or cirrhosis, may be seen in some patients, particularly those with hepatitis B.[66, 300] Progressive deterioration of renal function has also been noted.[104, 300] Antihistamines are effective in controlling an urticarial component that may rarely be present. Plasmapheresis has also been suggested as a possible therapeutic modality,[301] although it is not uniformly successful. Corticosteroid and immunosuppressive therapy is not of proven efficacy[105] but should be considered in patients with progressive renal dysfunction. On an individual basis, agents such as penicillamine[302] and epsilon-aminocaproic acid,[303] which increase the solubility of selected cryoglobulins, could theoretically be of benefit.

HYPERSENSITIVITY VASCULITIS ASSOCIATED WITH SYSTEMIC DISEASES

Introduction. Frequently, a pattern of hypersensitivity vasculitis is associated with a primary and underlying systemic disease, for example, a connective tissue disease, an autoimmune disease, or a malignancy. The hypersensitivity vasculitis seen in patients with an associated systemic disease appears to result from a reaction directed against endogenous antigens such as DNA, autologous immunoglobulins, and, possibly, tumor antigens. This response to endogenous antigens is in contrast to the allergic response in hypersensitivity vasculitis not associated with an underlying systemic disease, in which the abnormal immune response is directed toward an exogenous antigen.

Vasculitis associated with connective tissue disorders. Necrotizing vasculitis in a variable degree is seen in rheumatoid arthritis, SLE, Sjögren's syndrome, dermatomyositis, scleroderma, and rheumatic fever.[4, 214, 238, 304] Frequently, the hypersensitivity response can be traced to an endogenous antigen, such as a serum protein or DNA. The vasculitis may involve the small vessels of the skin with a pattern of hypersensitivity vasculitis. Less frequently, muscular arteries can be involved, producing a pattern of systemic necrotizing vasculitis as discussed in Chapter 4.

The two connective tissue diseases with the most frequent vasculitic involvement are rheumatoid arthritis and SLE.[304] The vasculitic component of rheumatoid arthritis is well established.[305, 306] Circulating immune complexes have been demonstrated in the serum of patients with this disease.[98] Patients with rheumatoid arthritis who develop vasculitis are more likely to have severe erosive joint disease,[307] hypocomplementemia,[308] circulating cryoglobulins,[309] and low molecular weight (7S) IgM.[310]

The most common pattern of vasculitis in rheumatoid arthritis is a leukocytoclastic venulitis of the skin[311] or the synovium or early rheumatoid nodules.[70] Patients usually present with palpable purpura without evidence of vasculitis elsewhere. Rarely, patients may develop a pattern of systemic necrotizing vasculitis that is clinically and histopathologically similar to PAN.[127, 306] Multiple organ system involvement may result in life-threatening visceral infarction (see Chapter 4). Originally, it was felt that corticosteroid therapy could precipitate or exacerbate rheumatoid vasculitis.[127, 312] However, it appears that patients with severe rheumatoid arthritis are more likely to develop vasculitis whether or not they receive corticosteroid therapy.[304]

Vasculitis in SLE may be present in variable degrees. Circulating immune complexes are common in SLE. Deposition of immunoglobulin and complement has been demonstrated in the skin[238] as well as other organ systems.[313] Approximately 20 per cent of patients with SLE will exhibit cutaneous vasculitis at some point in the disease. The lesions present as purpuric papules, which occur most commonly in the lower extremities but may be seen in any location, including the finger tips. Progression to chronic ulceration or gangrene of the digit is less frequent. Diffuse central nervous system vasculitis as well as a visceral vasculitis similar to PAN occurs less commonly.[313, 314]

Treatment should be directed at the underlying disease, whether it is rheumatoid arthritis or SLE. Corticosteroids may improve the vasculitis in some patients, but the response is variable. Although corticosteroids do not precipitate rheumatoid vasculitis,[304] necrotizing vasculitis may develop in patients with rheumatoid arthritis on corticosteroid therapy. In cases of systemic necrotizing vasculitis, particularly of the PAN type, a trial of immunosuppressive therapy such as cyclophosphamide (1 to 2 mg per kg per day) should be considered, based on the response to this drug in the systemic necrotizing vasculitic group of diseases (see Chapter 4). Proof of therapeutic efficacy awaits further studies.

Hypersensitivity vasculitis associated with malignancy. Vasculitis can occur in association with certain malignancies. It can be seen particularly with lymphoid or reticuloendothelial neoplasms, such as chronic lymphocytic leukemia, lymphoma, Hodgkin's disease, and multiple myeloma.[239, 315, 316] Cutaneous purpural lesions that demonstrate a leukocytoclastic pattern on biopsy are the most common finding. The spectrum of vasculitides associated with malignancy, which rarely includes a visceral vasculitis, is discussed in Chapter 9.

Vasculitis associated with other primary disorders. A leukocytoclastic vasculitis may be a minor component of a wide variety of other diseases.[238] Such diseases include subacute bacterial endocarditis, chronic active hepatitis, ulcerative colitis, retroperitoneal fibrosis, primary biliary cirrhosis, and Goodpasture's syndrome. An association between α_1-antitrypsin deficiency,[317] intestinal bypass surgery,[318] relapsing polychondritis,[319] and hypersensitivity vasculitis has also been suggested.

CHAPTER 6

WEGENER'S GRANULOMATOSIS

Definition.   Wegener's granulomatosis is a disease of unknown etiology characterized by a clinicopathologic complex of a necrotizing, granulomatous vasculitis of the upper and lower respiratory tracts, glomerulonephritis, and variable degrees of small vessel vasculitis.[7-9, 320]

Historical perspective.   Klinger[6] in 1931 reported the first case of the disease, but Wegener, in two publications in 1936 and 1939, established it as a distinct clinicopathologic entity.[7, 8] In 1954 detailed clinical[320] and pathologic[321] descriptions defined the diagnostic criteria for Wegener's granulomatosis. A limited form of Wegener's granulomatosis characterized by the absence of glomerular disease was described in 1966.[10] Confirmation of the observation that cytotoxic therapy markedly improved the prognosis in Wegener's granulomatosis was instrumental in the institution of cytotoxic therapy for certain non-neoplastic diseases.[9, 322-326]

Incidence and prevalence.   Wegener's granulomatosis is an uncommon disease. It is difficult to determine the true incidence and prevalence, although several hundred cases have been reported. The mean age of patients in the NIH series[9, 327] is just over 40 years. Although the greatest number of cases present in the fourth and fifth decades, the disease has been seen at both extremes of age. There is a slight male predominance with a ratio of approximately 3 to 2.

Pathophysiology.   Although the cause of Wegener's granulomatosis is unknown, the observation that the primary clinical involvement was in the respiratory tract[320, 321] suggested the possibility of an inhaled antigen or pathogen. However, attempts to demonstrate an infectious agent or an environmental antigen have been uniformly unsuccessful.

72

Although an inciting antigen has not been demonstrated, there is ample evidence for hyperreactivity of the immune system. Elevation of IgG and IgA with normal or slightly depressed IgM is characteristic of the disease.[9] The majority of patients will have low titers of rheumatoid factor in their serum. Studies in our laboratory have demonstrated increased B cell activity as measured by increased numbers of circulating B cells spontaneously secreting immunoglobulin (Cupps TR, Fauci AS, unpublished observation).

Despite the evident immune hyperreactivity as well as the presence of circulating immune complexes in certain patients, the exact role of circulating and deposited immune complexes is not clear[328] (Fauci AS, Lawley TJ, Frank MM, unpublished observation). Serum complement levels are generally not depressed. Electron microscopy studies in renal biopsies from patients with Wegener's granulomatosis have demonstrated immune complex–like material in only two of seven specimens despite an extensive evaluation.[329] Immunofluorescent studies have demonstrated IgG and complement in some,[9] but not all, cases.[95] Attempts to demonstrate immune complexes in lung and skin have also been unsuccessful.[95] Obviously, these relatively negative results must be cautiously interpreted in light of the rapid clearance of antigenic material from sites of active vasculitis (see Chapter 2). Nonetheless, pathophysiologic mechanisms other than immune complex deposition may well play a major role in this disease.

Studies of mononuclear cell function in Wegener's granulomatosis have demonstrated relatively normal function. The numbers of peripheral blood lymphocytes, monocytes, T cells, and B cells tend to be normal.[9, 330] In general, responses to skin-test antigens and blastogenic responses to mitogens such as concanavalin A and phytohemagglutinin are normal.[9, 330] Recent observations,[328, 331] suggesting abnormalities in lymphocyte function, are difficult to interpret because treated patients, as well as patients with other diseases such as midline granuloma, were inclined in the study.

Recent studies[332, 333] suggest a possible abnormality of polymorphonuclear function in patients with Wegener's granulomatosis. Electron microscopy studies of a lung biopsy of a patient with limited Wegener's granulomatosis[332] are reported to have shown intravascular lysis of leukocytes as an early event in the inflammatory process. The significance of this observation is unclear. A chemotactic abnormality has also been suggested.[333] However, interpretation of this observation is difficult because treated patients as well as individuals who may not have had Wegener's granulomatosis were included in the study group. Further evaluation of these preliminary observations should be pursued.

The etiology of the renal lesion in Wegener's granulomatosis deserves further consideration. As previously noted, convincing evi-

TABLE 6-1. FREQUENCY OF PRESENTING COMPLAINTS IN
PATIENTS WITH WEGENER'S GRANULOMATOSIS°

PRESENTING PROBLEM	PERCENTAGE
Head and neck	85
Sinusitis/nasal obstruction	53
Ear (otitis, hearing loss, pain)	15
Gingival inflammation	6
Epistaxis	6
Sore throat/laryngitis	5
"Saddle nose" deformity	4
Lower respiratory tract	34
Cough/sputum production	16
Dyspnea	8
Pleurisy/chest pain	6
Hemoptysis	4
Fever	12
Extremity involvement	9
Arthralgia	4
Arthritis	2
Extremity pain	2
Myalgias	1
Weight loss	5
Headache	5
Malaise/weakness	4
Orchitis	2
Skin lesions	2

°Data are summarized from 85 patients reviewed in references 320 and 336.
Multiple symptoms were recorded for the majority of patients.

dence for immune complex deposition in renal biopsies can be
found in only a minority of patients.[329] In one patient[334] there was
no evidence of immune complex deposition on renal biopsy by
immunofluorescence or electron microscopy, despite the presence
of circulating immune complexes. Only fibrin could be demonstrated by immunofluorescence. Intracapillary clotting preceded rapidly
progressive glomerulonephritis in another patient with Wegener's
granulomatosis.[335] The significance of these observations with respect to the renal lesion and the pathophysiology of the disease as a
whole is not well defined.

Clinical manifestations. The presenting signs and symptoms of
85 patients with Wegener's granulomatosis[320, 336] are summarized in
Table 6-1. The great majority of patients present with problems
related to the upper respiratory tract. Symptoms of sinusitis, rhinitis, nasal obstruction, and problems related to the ears, such as otitis
media, pain, and decreased hearing, are most common. Less frequently, complaints are related to the head and neck region and

include gingival inflammation, epistaxis, sore throat or laryngitis, and "saddle nose" deformity. Signs and symptoms related to the lower respiratory tract are noted in a third of patients and include cough and sputum production, dyspnea, chest pain, and hemoptysis.

Even less frequently presenting complaints are limited to non-specific findings such as fever, myalgias, arthralgias, and weight loss. Rarely, patients may present with skin lesions or orchitis. Of particular interest, symptoms related to the urinary tract and gastro-intestinal tract are generally absent.

Several unusual presentations deserve further comment. Skin lesions can predate other systemic manifestations by months.[337] When skin lesions are the initial findings, the lesions usually have a distinctive appearance of "punched-out" ulcers characteristic of pyoderma gangrenosum.[337] Moreover, presenting skin lesions, including painful subcutaneous nodules, have been reported to be more common in the limited form of Wegener's granulomatosis.[10, 338]

The frequency of organ system involvement summarized in Table 6–2 reflects our own experience with Wegener's granulomatosis at the National Institutes of Health.

LUNG. Although symptomatic pulmonary manifestations are present in only a third of patients, evidence for lung involvement is seen in essentially all patients after a complete evaluation. Even in the absence of symptoms related to the chest, chest roentgenograms are frequently abnormal. Cough, dyspnea, and chest pain are the most frequent symptoms. Hemoptysis is seen less frequently. Rarely, massive life-threatening pulmonary hemorrhage mimicking Goodpasture's syndrome may be seen.[9, 339]

PARANASAL SINUSES. Clinical involvement of the paranasal sinuses as well as abnormal sinus roentgenograms is present in nearly all patients. Symptoms of acute sinusitis, rhinitis, or nasal obstruction may be present. The most frequently involved sinuses

TABLE 6–2. *FREQUENCY OF ORGAN SYSTEM INVOLVEMENT IN PATIENTS WITH WEGENER'S GRANULOMATOSIS**

ORGAN SYSTEM	PERCENTAGE
Lungs	100
Paranasal sinuses	95
Nasopharynx	91
Urinary tract	81
Joints	57
Skin	48
Eyes	43
Ears	38
Heart	29
Nervous system	24

*Table summarizes information from 21 patients reviewed in reference 327.

are the maxillary (68 per cent), sphenoid (28 per cent), and eth-moids (14 per cent).[340] The underlying disease may be complicated by a superimposed bacterial infection, particularly with *Staphylo-coccus aureus.*

NASOPHARYNX. Inflammatory or vasculitic lesions or both can be present at any site in the upper airways. Destruction of the cartilage of the nasal septum results in the "saddle nose" deformity. Oral lesions tend to be shallow ulcers with sharp margins, and a persistent sore throat may be the major complaint.[341] Through-and-through perforation of the hard or soft palate is virtually never seen in Wegener's granulomatosis.[9] If such a lesion is present, another diagnosis, such as midline granuloma,[342] should be considered.

Gingivitis with granulomatous inflammation has also been de-scribed and may precede evidence of systemic involvement by months.[343-346] Additional findings include bleeding from the gingival margins, loss of teeth, resorption of alveolar bone, and delayed healing following a tooth extraction.

URINARY TRACT. From a clinical standpoint, the renal in-volvement is usually asymptomatic at presentation. After a complete evaluation, however, evidence of renal involvement is seen in 80 per cent of cases, generally in the form of an abnormal urinary sediment.[327] Functional impairment may also be present initially and may progress rapidly in the absence of appropriate therapeutic intervention.[9] Rarely, a picture of perinephric hematoma[200] or ure-teral vasculitis with secondary obstruction is seen.[347] As opposed to systemic necrotizing vasculitis, hypertension associated with renal involvement is the exception rather than the rule.

JOINTS. Symptomatic joints are present in over half the pa-tients with Wegener's granulomatosis. Arthralgias are much more common than true arthritis, with a tendency toward multijoint in-volvement. Progression to destructive joint deformities has not been described. Rarely, the presence of arthritis may precede the onset of systemic symptoms by several months.[348]

TABLE 6-3.   *CUTANEOUS INVOLVEMENT IN WEGENER'S GRANULOMATOSIS**

	PERCENTAGE OF	
LESION	CUTANEOUS LESIONS	PATIENTS WITH LESIONS
Ulceration	75	33
Papules	37	17
Vesicles	12	6
Subcutaneous nodules	12	6

*Data summarize experience of 8 of 18 patients reported in reference 9. Three of eight patients had more than one type of cutaneous lesion.

Skin. We have recently reviewed the cutaneous manifestations of Wegener's granulomatosis.[349] Cutaneous lesions are found in 40 to 50 per cent of patients.[9, 336, 350] The frequency of various skin lesions is summarized in Table 6–3. The most common lesions are ulcerative (75 per cent) and papular (37 per cent). Less frequently, vesicles, petechiae, and subcutaneous nodules are reported. Other unusual cutaneous manifestations include nonhealing of surgical wounds[351] and necrosis of the penis.[352]

Eye. The eye manifestations of Wegener's granulomatosis have been reviewed in detail[340] and are summarized in Table 6–4. Ocular involvement may be a presenting symptom.[340] The most common finding is proptosis followed by inflammation of the anterior structures of the eye. Vasculitis of the optic vessels is seen in 10 per cent of cases. Failure to rapidly initiate appropriate therapy in patients with eye involvement may result in rapid functional impairment. The corneal degeneration secondary to occlusive vasculitis[352] can be corrected by corneal transplant after the underlying inflammatory process has been controlled with appropriate medical therapy.[353, 354]

Ear. The most common finding related to the ear is otitis media secondary to obstruction of the eustachian tubes. Less frequently, primary involvement of auricular structures with a granulomatous inflammation is seen,[9] with resultant otorrhea, decreased hearing, and ear pain. Auricular chondritis has also been described in a case of Wegener's granulomatosis.[355]

Heart. Any structure in the heart may be involved in Wegener's granulomatosis.[321, 336, 356, 357] Pericarditis is the most common clinical manifestation; involvement of the endocardium including the valves has been reported,[356, 357] as have pancarditis and coronary artery vasculitis.[9, 336, 356, 357] Intractable cardiac arrhythmias, presumably secondary to vasculitis-induced ischemia, have also been noted.[9]

TABLE 6–4. *OCULAR MANIFESTATIONS IN WEGENER'S GRANULOMATOSIS* *

Manifestation	Percentage†	Number of Observations‡
Ocular involvement	39	371
Proptosis	19	315
Conjunctivitis, episcleritis, scleritis, corneoscleral ulcer	17	315
Optic nerve vasculitis	9	315
Nasolacrimal duct disease	3	315
Uveitis	2	315

*Data are summarized from a literature review detailed in reference 340.
†Per cent involvement of patients with Wegener's granulomatosis.
‡Number of patients for whom a given manifestation was evaluated.

NERVOUS SYSTEM. Dysfunction of the nervous system can be seen in 25 per cent of patients.[327] The most common site of involvement is the peripheral nervous system, with a pattern of mononeuritis multiplex or polyneuritis.[358] Involvement of the structures at the base of the brain, including the pituitary and cranial nerves (particularly the optic and auditory nerves), secondary to a contiguous spread from the inflammatory process of the nasal or paranasal structures is not uncommon.[358] Less frequently, a central nervous system vasculitis with or without associated subarachnoid or intracerebral hemorrhage is seen.[358] Diabetes insipidus, felt to be secondary to central nervous system involvement, has been reported.[359]

Limited form of Wegener's granulomatosis. The concept of a limited form of Wegener's granulomatosis was initially suggested by Carrington and Liebow.[10] They identified a group of patients with the diagnostic criterion for Wegener's granulomatosis in the absence of renal glomerular lesions. This group of patients was characterized by a better prognosis (although fatal cases were described) and by an apparent responsiveness to corticosteroid therapy.[10] Subsequent authors could not confirm responsiveness to the steroid therapy.[338] Interestingly, the most frequent presenting signs or symptoms are related to the lower respiratory tract with notable absence of upper respiratory tract symptoms.[10, 338] More frequent cutaneous involvement, particularly with ulcers or subcutaneous nodules, has already been noted.

It is likely that a number of cases that have been considered as limited Wegener's granulomatosis were in fact the generalized form with subclinical and undetected renal diseases. This possibility was highlighted by us in our initial reported series of patients,[9] in which renal biopsies were performed on all patients with Wegener's granulomatosis regardless of the presence or absence of clinically detectable renal disease. It was demonstrated that over 50 per cent of patients with presumed limited Wegener's granulomatosis indeed had the generalized form, since their renal biopsy demonstrated focal glomerulonephritis, despite the lack of clinically apparent renal disease.

Laboratory considerations. There are no laboratory tests that reveal an abnormality diagnostic of Wegener's granulomatosis. However, abnormalities of certain rather nonspecific laboratory determinations are characteristic of the disease. The erythrocyte sedimentation rate is invariably elevated in active Wegener's granulomatosis. Extreme elevations to greater than 100 mm per hour are usually seen. The majority of patients have a leukocytosis with or without increased numbers of band forms. Thrombocytosis is frequently present, reflecting acute-phase reactants. Leukopenia or thrombocytopenia in an untreated patient is quite rare. Hyperreactivity of the immune system is suggested by elevated immunoglobulins.[9] Elevation of IgG and IgA is present in the majority of patients. The IgM fraction may be normal or slightly depressed. An elevation of IgE has been described[93, 94] but has not been confirmed by all the authors.[95] Rheumatoid factor is present in 60 per cent of patients. Cryoglobulins can be demonstrated in only a minority of patients. Circulating immune complexes are present in some, but not all, patients with active untreated Wegener's granulomatosis. Abnormal urinary sediment is present in 80 per cent of patients.[9] Hematuria, with or without red blood cell casts, together with proteinuria is the most common pattern. Proteinuria may be extensive, approaching a pattern of nephrotic syndrome. Rapid deterioration of renal function with oliguria or even anuria may be seen in patients with untreated Wegener's granulomatosis.

Radiographic studies can provide important information in patients with this disease. The findings on roentgenograms of the chest have been reviewed in detail (Fig. 6–1).[9, 360, 361] Table 6–5 summarizes the experience in this regard at the National Institutes of Health.[362] The "typical" finding is multiple, nodular, bilateral, cavitary infiltrates. However, single or multiple lesions may be present. Infiltrates without a sharply defined margin are more frequent than discrete nodular lesions (Table 6–5). Cavitation is seen in both kinds of lesions and is either unilocular or multilocular with irregular margins.[360, 361] The cavities have been described as thick-walled,[361] but some authors[360] maintain that thin-walled cavities are

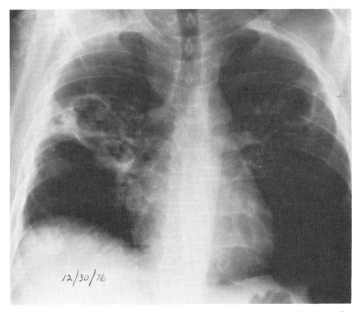

12/30/76

Figure 6–1. Chest x-ray film from a patient with Wegener's granulomatosis. Multiple cavitary lung lesions are seen bilaterally in the midlung fields.

*TABLE 6–5. SUMMARY OF CHEST ROENTGENOGRAPHIC FINDINGS IN PATIENTS WITH WEGENER'S GRANULOMATOSIS**

FINDING	PERCENTAGE
Distribution	
Unilateral	54
Bilateral	46
Lesion	
Infiltrate	52
Cavitation	10
Nodule	27
Cavitation	7

*Data are summarized from chest films reviewed in 41 patients reported in reference 362.

more common and that a false appearance of a thin cavity wall is given in a plain roentgenogram because the surrounding lung is often infiltrated. Infiltrates may be present in the upper and lower lung fields and may be transient in nature.[9, 360] Narrowing of the bronchial lumen may be seen as a result of active endobronchial disease or scarring secondary to previously active disease. Unusual findings on routine chest radiographs in patients with Wegener's granulomatosis include a mass between the trachea and esophagus, calcified nodule, paratracheal mass, large cavity lesions, miliary pattern suggestive of tuberculosis, and massive pleural effusion.[363] Sinus films are abnormal in the majority of patients, reflecting the frequent involvement in this area.[9] Findings range from mucosal thickening to pansinusitis with multiple air-fluid levels.

Less commonly, other radiographic studies are abnormal. Although intravenous pyelograms are generally normal in this disease, rarely, an irregular pattern along the ureter with or without obstructions will suggest the diagnosis of vasculitis.[347] Rare findings on renal angiograms include demonstration of aneurysms[200] and definition of vascular inflammatory masses.[363]

Computer-assisted tomography may be of value in determining ocular involvement in this disease.[340, 364] Involvement of the retro-orbital space may result from an extension of an inflammatory process from an adjacent structure, or it may reflect a primary retro-orbital process. Serial orbital computer-assisted tomographic studies may help to evaluate a patient with an acute deterioration of vision. If a rapidly expanding retro-orbital mass is defined, surgical intervention or treatment for an infectious process or both should be considered. In the absence of an expanding lesion, the change in vision is probably related to a vascular lesion and surgical intervention is not indicated.

Pathology. The hallmark of Wegener's granulomatosis is a necrotizing granulomatous vasculitis (Fig. 6–2).[321] The vasculitis is

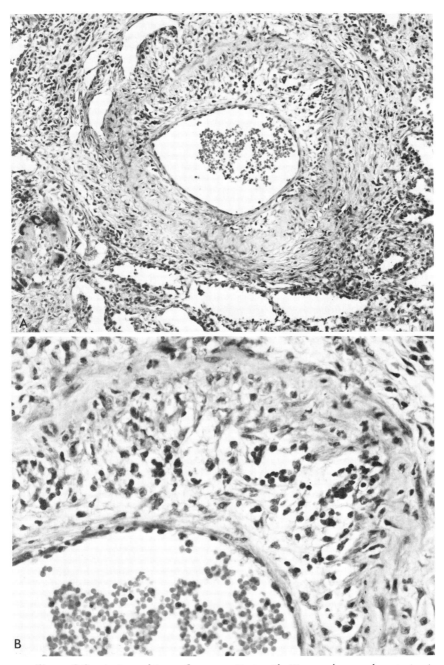

Figure 6–2. A, Lung biopsy from a patient with Wegener's granulomatosis. A necrotizing vasculitis and adjacent multinucleated giant cells (lower left) are seen. Hematoxylin and eosin stain (original magnification ×130). *B*, A more detailed view of the vessel seen in A. There is a mixed cellular infiltrate of the vessel wall, although mononuclear cells predominate. Hematoxylin and eosin stain (original magnification ×330).

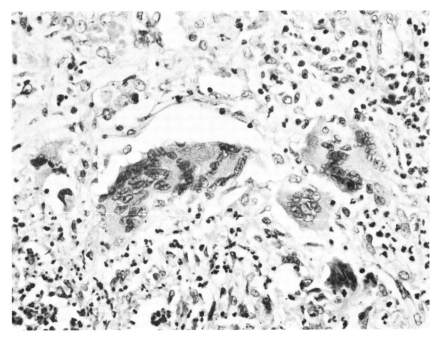

Figure 6–3. Lung biopsy from a patient with Wegener's granulomatosis. A cluster of multinucleated giant cells is seen adjacent to an area of necrosis. Hematoxylin and eosin stain (original magnification ×330).

predominantly a fibrinoid necrosis of small arteries and veins with early infiltration of polymorphonuclear leukocytes followed by mononuclear cells and healing with fibrosis. All stages of lesions may be present at a given time. Granulomata are usually well formed with plentiful giant cells (Fig. 6–3). The granuloma may be within, adjacent to, or spatially dissociated from the vascular lesion. Large areas of necrosis may be seen, particularly in the lung. These may be directly associated with the granuloma formation or may result from vasculitis-related ischemia.

Although involvement of the upper respiratory tract, lower respiratory tract, and kidneys is characteristic, essentially any organ system can be affected (Table 6–2).[321] Any combination of granuloma, vasculitis, and necrosis may be present at a given site.

The renal lesions can be quite variable.[9, 321, 329] The most common pattern of renal disease is a focal and segmental glomerulonephritis. A pattern of diffuse proliferative glomerulonephritis with crescent formation may be seen with rapidly deteriorating renal function. Basement membrane crimping and increased mesangial material along the capillary wall also occurs.[329] Less frequently, vasculitis, granuloma formation, or a pattern of interstitial nephritis can be seen. Electron microscopy studies on renal biopsies may demonstrate subepithelial basement membrane densities, suggesting immune complex deposition. This finding, however, can be demonstrated in only a minority of cases.

Diagnosis and differential diagnosis. Wegener's granulomatosis is a clinicopathologic diagnosis. The diagnosis is established in an appropriate clinical setting when a biopsy demonstrates the characteristic necrotizing granulomatous vasculitis.[9] The biopsy site most likely to have the characteristic pathologic findings is the lung. In general, the tissue sample from a transbronchial biopsy will be inadequate; consequently, an open lung biopsy done through a limited thoracotomy is generally preferred and is well tolerated by most patients.[9, 327] Although biopsies from active sites in the nasopharynx may show the characteristic histopathology, frequently a pattern of chronic inflammation with or without granuloma will only suggest the diagnosis. Less frequently, the typical histopathologic features may be present on biopsies from the retro-orbital area, auditory canal, skin, or muscle.

Because sites other than the lung may be biopsied first, interpretation of the results with respect to the diagnosis and management of Wegener's granulomatosis deserves further comment. The finding of a focal and segmental glomerulonephritis with or without granuloma in the appropriate clinical setting should suggest the diagnosis. Furthermore, renal biopsy may be helpful in defining the extent of disease. Some patients thought to have the limited form of disease because of a normal renal function and a relatively normal urinary sediment may manifest early focal glomerular involvement on biopsy.[9] The finding of glomerulonephritis can help exclude such diseases as lymphomatoid granulomatosis (see Chapter 7) and midline granuloma[342] from the differential diagnosis. Finally, the renal biopsy can provide useful prognostic information regarding eventual renal function. Patients with acute renal function impairment with an active inflammatory process in the glomeruli are more likely to have a significant return of function following appropriate therapy than if most glomeruli are sclerosed.

Because of easy access, skin biopsies are frequently done. Although a pattern of granulomatous inflammation or necrotizing granuloma can suggest the diagnosis, a necrotizing granulomatous vasculitis will be present in only a minority of skin biopsy specimens.[349] Nondiagnostic patterns of chronic inflammation and leukocytoclastic vasculitis are commonly seen[9, 349]; panniculitis has also been reported.[365]

As noted in Table 6–1, gingival disease may be a presenting complaint and periodontal disease may precede systemic signs of Wegener's granulomatosis by months.[346, 366] Biopsies of gingival tissue may show granulomata with acute and chronic inflammation but without vasculitis. This pattern, however, is so unusual in other diseases that it is highly suggestive of the diagnosis of Wegener's granulomatosis in the appropriate clinical setting.[346]

The differential diagnosis can include a large number of disease processes, depending on the clinical presentation.[9, 327] Diseases with a *predominantly vasculitic picture*, such as systemic necrotizing vasculitis, systemic lupus erythematosus, scleroderma, dermatomyositis, Sjögren's syndrome, Henoch-Schönlein purpura, and hypersensitivity vasculitis, must be excluded. *Granulomatous diseases*, such as sarcoidosis, berylliosis, and midline granuloma, are not associated with a necrotizing vasculitis. *Mixed granulomatous and vasculitic diseases* can closely mimic the clinical presentation of Wegener's granulomatosis. Allergic angiitis and granulomatosis are characterized by a necrotizing granulomatous vasculitis of pulmonary vessels. Unlike Wegener's granulomatosis, blood eosinophilia, tissue infiltration with eosinophils, and an allergic history are characteristic of this disease. In this regard, several diseases that produce infiltrates and eosinophilia may have granulomata and vasculitis as part of their histologic picture. Included in this latter group are neoplastic, parasitic, allergic, and connective tissue diseases. Lymphomatoid granulomatosis is a disease characterized by an angiocentric, angioinvasive, and angiodestructive infiltration of vessels with atypical lymphoid and plasmacytoid cells (see Chapter 7). Renal parenchyma may be infiltrated by these atypical cells, but renal glomeruli are not involved primarily in this disease process.

Infectious granulomatous diseases. Diseases such as tuberculosis, histoplasmosis, blastomycosis, coccidioidomycosis, and syphilis can be excluded by appropriate cultures, special stains, and serologic studies. *Pulmonary-renal syndromes* such as Goodpasture's syndrome and streptococcal pneumonia with glomerulonephritis must also be excluded. Goodpasture's syndrome, which presents with pulmonary hemorrhage and glomerulonephritis,[367] can be identified by the demonstration of antiglomerular basement membrane antibody.[368, 369] Streptococcal pneumonia is excluded by appropriate cultures and serologic studies. *Neoplastic diseases* (including nasopharyngeal carcinomas, lymphomas and sarcomas, primary and metastatic lung tumors, Hodgkin's disease, and lymphoma of the lung) may have a granulomatous reaction. The presence of neoplastic cells in the inflammatory lesion, however, establishes the diagnosis of a neoplastic process.

Treatment and prognosis. Untreated Wegener's granulomatosis has a mean survival of 5 months with a 90 per cent mortality rate at 2 years.[336] The use of corticosteroids has improved this bleak prognosis only modestly.[370] It is noteworthy that cytotoxic agents have induced clinical remissions in a high proportion of patients.[9, 322-326] Clearly, cyclophosphamide is the most effective agent[9, 322, 371, 372] and is the drug of choice in patients with Wegener's granulomatosis and renal involvement. Generally, the drug is started at 1 to 2 mg per kg per day orally. For rapidly progressive renal disease, 2 to 4 mg per kg per day may be given intravenously for the initial 3 to 4 days before returning to the standard dose. Higher doses increase the risk of granulocytopenia without improving the immunosuppressive effect of the drug[327] and should be avoided. After the initial week of therapy, the white blood cell count is followed to titrate the dose of cyclophosphamide for each individual. Care should be taken to avoid suppressing the total white blood cell count below 3000 cells/mm^3 or a polymorphonuclear leukocyte count below 1500 cells/mm^3. Treatment should be continued through a minimum of a 1-year disease-free interval before attempts to withdraw the drug are considered. Close follow-up for reactivation during this period is indicated. If the disease reactivates, a second course of cyclophosphamide is generally effective in producing a sustained clinical remission. Sustained remissions seen in over 90 per cent of patients treated with cyclophosphamide have been reported.[327, 371]

Immunosuppressive agents other than cyclophosphamide have been recommended for the treatment of Wegener's granulomatosis. In particular, Israel and Patchefsky[326, 373] suggest the use of chlorambucil in the limited form of Wegener's, citing an increased incidence of complications with cyclophosphamide. Care must be exercised if this agent is used, because renal involvement by biopsy can be demonstrated in the presence of a normal urinary sediment.[9] Because cyclophosphamide is of proven efficacy and the drug can be used relatively safely with appropriate monitoring of the leukocyte count,[330] we consider it the initial drug of choice in all patients with Wegener's granulomatosis.[374]

If complications of therapy, such as severe cystitis, develop (see Chapter 15), alternative cytotoxic agents such as azathioprine or chlorambucil can be used. Although cyclophosphamide is clearly superior in inducing remissions in active Wegener's granulomatosis, these latter agents (particularly azathioprine) have proved effective in maintaining remission in certain patients whose disease was put into remission with cyclophosphamide, but in whom cyclophosphamide had to be discontinued because of adverse side effects, particularly cystitis.

Corticosteroids are an important adjunct to cytotoxic therapy. Generally prednisone, 1 mg per kg per day orally in single or divided doses, is started with cyclophosphamide. After 10 days to 2 weeks, when the immunosuppressive effects of the cyclophosphamide become apparent, the prednisone dose regimen is consolidated to a single daily dose, tapered rapidly to an alternate-day regimen, and ultimately discontinued, depending on the individual clinical response. Severe pulmonary, renal, or skin disease may benefit from more prolonged courses of corticosteroid therapy together with cyclophosphamide.[327] Severe serosal surface involvement, such as pericarditis, may benefit from a more aggressive therapy with prednisone initially. Rheumatic symptoms such as arthritis or vasculitic skin rash may occur despite adequate immunosuppression with cyclophosphamide. These symptoms respond rapidly to a short burst of daily corticosteroid therapy followed by a rapid taper to an alternate-day regimen. Some patients will continue to have evidence of low-grade disease activity, despite a total leukocyte count of 3000 cells/mm³. The addition of alternate-day prednisone to such a regimen for its granulopoietic sparing effect[375] frequently allows increased doses of cyclophosphamide to be used safely.

Serious eye involvement is an absolute indication for corticosteroid therapy regardless of whether the other systemic manifestations are well controlled on cytotoxic agents.[340] The corticosteroid regimen (usually prednisone, 1 mg per kg per day) should be continued until ocular disease activity subsides, at which point the steroid is gradually tapered to an alternate-day regimen and ultimately discontinued.

With the successful treatment of Wegener's granulomatosis, long-term management considerations have become important. The erythrocyte sedimentation rate, in general, reflects disease activity. In several patients it has taken up to 1 year to normalize. An elevation of a previously normalized sedimentation rate well into the course of immunosuppressive therapy may be caused by an underlying disease flare-up or, more commonly, by intercurrent infection such as a bacterial sinusitis. Moreover, proteinuria may persist despite adequate control of the renal disease and is generally not associated with a progressive decline in renal function.

Frequently, patients with Wegener's granulomatosis sustain irreversible damage to the paranasal sinuses; consequently, long-term local mucosal care is required. Commonly, drainage procedures will be required because of recurrent bacterial infections, despite control of the inflammatory process. Local irrigation with saline may also be useful.

Obstruction of the large airways can be a difficult management problem.[362] Four of 47 patients followed at the National Institutes of Health developed this problem. The most common site of obstruction, seen in three of the patients, was the subglottic region. Generally the problem responds to dilatation when the underlying inflammatory disease is under control.[362] One patient, however, required resection of a stenotic region of the left main stem bronchus. Local radiotherapy has been suggested for stenotic areas that show evidence of inflammatory activity despite apparently adequate cyclophosphamide therapy.[376]

If the diagnosis and institution of appropriate therapy are delayed, patients may proceed to chronic renal failure. Renal transplantation can be successfully done in patients with Wegener's granulomatosis while in clinical remission.[377] Of interest, a recurrence of the Wegener's granulomatosis in a transplanted kidney was reported despite therapy with azathioprine.[378] Reinduction with cyclophosphamide was successful, further confirming the greater efficacy of cyclophosphamide in this disease as compared with other cytotoxic agents.

CHAPTER 7

LYMPHOMATOID GRANULOMATOSIS

Definition. Lymphomatoid granulomatosis, an unusual granulomatous vasculitis initially described by Liebow and colleagues in 1972,[11] is characterized by a multisystemic, angiocentric, angiodestructive infiltration with atypical lymphocytoid and plasmacytoid cells.

Incidence and prevalence. Lymphomatoid granulomatosis is a rare disease, with fewer than 200 cases reported since its description. A review of 161 cases[95, 379] shows a mean age at onset of 48 years with a range of 7 to 85 years, and a slight male to female preponderance of 1.6 to 1.

Pathophysiology. The etiology of lymphomatoid granulomatosis is unknown, and there is no evidence to suggest a primary role for immune complex–mediated vascular damage. The pattern of a cellular infiltrate with predominantly mononuclear cells and an extravascular cellular infiltrate argues against immune complex–mediated disease. Tests of cellular immunity, including intradermal skin testing with recall antigens, dinitrochlorobenzene skin sensitization, and response to phytohemagglutinin, may be abnormal.[380] It remains unclear whether lymphomatoid granulomatosis is a hypersensitivity disease that has neoplastic features or a primary neoplasm with an associated hypersensitivity reaction.[374]

The spectrum of lymphomatoid granulomatosis. Lymphomatoid granulomatosis[11] is a truly puzzling entity. Clearly, this disease comprises a spectrum ranging from a more benign form referred to as "benign lymphocytic angiitis and granulomatosis,"[95] to the more classic lymphomatoid granulomatosis that has not yet undergone malignant transformation, to a full-blown lymphoproliferative neoplasm that had originally manifested features of lymphomatoid gran-

88

ulomatosis or that persists in manifesting features of lymphomatoid granulomatosis despite the simultaneous presence of unequivocally neoplastic features. Patients who have progressed from "benign lymphocytic angiitis and granulomatosis" to lymphomatoid granulomatosis to frank lymphoma have been described and clearly documented.[374] Obvious difficulties arise in establishing the appropriate definitions as well as an orderly therapeutic approach to this disease given the complexity of the spectrum. Furthermore, since the disease may express itself in a benign form in one organ system such as the skin while simultaneously manifesting clear-cut lymphoma in another organ system such as the lung or the central nervous system (Fauci AS, unpublished observations), proper staging is a difficult task.

Clinical considerations. The presenting signs and symptoms of lymphomatoid granulomatosis are summarized in Table 7–1. Systemic symptoms, including fever, malaise, and weight loss, are frequently found. Respiratory symptoms, including cough, shortness of breath, and chest pain, are the most common focal findings. Neurologic dysfunction, including both peripheral neuropathies and CNS abnormalities, can be found in 21 per cent of patients. Less common presenting symptoms include cutaneous lesions, arthralgia, myalgia, and gastrointestinal distress. Three per cent of patients were asymptomatic. Of interest, the fever and neurologic symptoms may precede clinically apparent pulmonary involvement by months to years.[381-383]

Clinical involvement by organ system in lymphomatoid granulomatosis is summarized in Table 7–2.

PULMONARY. Lung involvement is characteristic of the disease. Cough and dyspnea are the most common symptoms. Pleuritic

TABLE 7–1. *PRESENTING SIGNS AND SYMPTOMS IN LYMPHOMATOID GRANULOMATOSIS**

PRESENTING SIGN OR SYMPTOM	PERCENTAGE
Fever	57
Cough	53
Malaise	35
Weight loss	34
Dyspnea	28
Neurologic dysfunction	21
Chest pain	13
Cutaneous lesion	11
Arthralgia	7
Myalgia	3
Gastrointestinal tract distress	3
Asymptomatic	3

*Data summarized from 161 patients reviewed in references 95 and 379.

TABLE 7–2. CLINICALLY APPARENT ORGAN SYSTEM
INVOLVEMENT IN LYMPHOMATOID GRANULOMATOSIS*

ORGAN SYSTEM INVOLVEMENT	PERCENTAGE
Pulmonary	100
Cutaneous	40
Neurologic	30
Central nervous system	19
Cranial neuropathy	11
Peripheral neuropathy	7
Splenomegaly	18
Hepatomegaly	12
Lymphadenopathy	8

*Data summarized from 161 patients reported in references 95 and 379.

or atypical chest pain is found less frequently. Hemoptysis is relatively rare but may be life-threatening.[11]

CUTANEOUS. Skin involvement at some time during the course of the disease is seen in 40 per cent of patients with lymphomatoid granulomatosis. Two kinds of lesions, erythematous macules and indurated plaque-like lesions, can be seen. The cutaneous involvement is most commonly seen in the lower extremities and the gluteal area, with less frequent involvement of the abdomen.[384]

NEUROLOGIC. Evidence of neurologic dysfunction is present in nearly a third of patients. CNS disease is the most common form of neurologic disease, potentially involving any site in the brain or brain stem. Cranial and peripheral neuropathies are less frequently observed.

VISCERAL. Splenomegaly, hepatomegaly, and lymphadenopathy are less often clinically apparent.

The most common cause of death in this disease is progressive pulmonary disease leading to respiratory insufficiency or, less frequently, to exsanguinating pulmonary hemorrhage.[380] This usually occurs in patients in whom the disease has undergone malignant transformation, although this may not be recognized at the time.

Uncontrolled CNS disease, which is the second most frequent cause of death, may be seen despite apparent control of pulmonary disease; infections, frequently associated with aggressive chemotherapy, may be a contributory cause of death.

Laboratory considerations. An elevated leukocyte count is seen in 50 per cent of patients, while leukopenia can be seen in 20 per cent.[379] A relative lymphocytosis, if present, may suggest progression to a frank neoplastic process.[11] The hematocrit is normal in the majority of patients. The erythrocyte sedimentation rate (ESR) is normal or minimally elevated in the majority of patients, and striking elevations of the ESR are characteristically not seen.[11] Immunoglobulins are normal in the majority of patients, although a mild polyclonal elevation will be present in some.

Evaluation of cerebral spinal fluid may be normal in nearly half the cases of lymphomatoid granulomatosis involving the CNS.[385, 386] Abnormalities of cerebral spinal fluid that have been described singly or in combination include elevated opening pressure, mildly elevated protein, mild pleocytosis, and the presence of "atypical" cells on cytopathologic evaluation.

Diagnostic radiologic studies, particularly the chest film, can provide useful information.[11, 95, 379] The most common pattern, generally present in the lower lung fields, consists of nodular densities in varying sizes (Fig. 7–1). The lesions are bilateral in nearly 80 per cent of cases.[379] The pattern is often strongly suggestive of metastatic tumor. Pleural effusions and cavitation are seen in 33 per cent and 30 per cent of cases, respectively, and hilar adenopathy is characteristically absent. Despite the presence of a parenchymal lesion adjacent to the pleura, there is generally minimal pleural reaction. Less frequently, an alveolar pattern or poorly defined "fluffy" infiltrate can be seen.[379] Cerebral angiography in the presence of CNS involvement may show a pattern of narrowing consistent with the diagnosis of angiitis[11] or, in some cases, findings consistent with a space-occupying mass lesion.

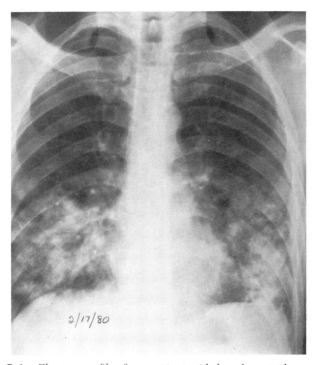

Figure 7–1. Chest x-ray film for a patient with lymphomatoid granulomatosis. Bilateral involvement of the lower lung fields as demonstrated in this film is the most common pattern in this disease.

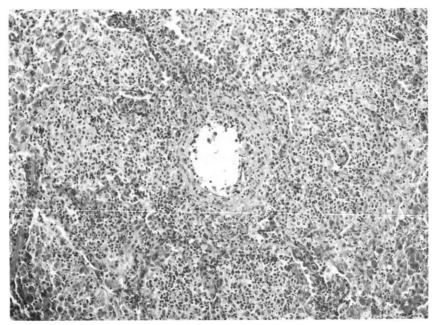

Figure 7–2. Lung biopsy from a patient with lymphomatoid granulomatosis. Note the mononuclear cell infiltrate around the vessels with invasion into the vascular wall producing the characteristic angiocentric, angiodestructive pattern. Hematoxylin and eosin stain (original magnification × 130).

Pathology. The characteristic histologic pattern seen in both veins and arteries is an angiocentric, angiodestructive inflammatory infiltrate of predominantly pleomorphic mononuclear cells with sparse granuloma formation.[11] The predominant cell pattern is a "lymphoid" or "plasmacytoid" cell with varying degrees of cellular atypia (Fig. 7–2). Electron microscopy studies support the apparent lymphoid origin of these cells.[387] Necrosis and mitotic figures are present to a variable degree. Histiocytic cells and eosinophils are less frequently seen. The degree of architectural destruction may be so severe that elastin stains may be required to demonstrate the remnant of a vessel in the center of an inflammatory mass.

The frequency of organ system involvement at autopsy is reviewed in Table 7–3. The most common site of involvement is the lung.[11] The second most frequent site, the kidney (Figs. 7–3 and 7–4), is of particular interest because disease involvement of this organ is seldom clinically apparent. Although the angiocentric, angiodestructive inflammatory pattern, including necrosis, can be seen in the kidney, a pleomorphic, mononuclear cell infiltrate in the interstitial space is the most common renal finding. The glomeruli are characteristically spared. Interestingly, despite major pathologic abnormalities, an evaluation of the urinary sediment may be entirely normal.[11, 379]

TABLE 7–3. ORGAN SYSTEM INVOLVEMENT IN LYMPHOMATOID GRANULOMATOSIS AT AUTOPSY*

ORGAN SYSTEM	PERCENTAGE
Lung	100
Kidney	32
Liver	29
Brain	26
Spleen	17
Adrenal gland	12
Heart	11

*Data summarized from 72 autopsies reviewed in reference 379. Note that skin evaluation was not routinely included in the postmortem studies.

Brain involvement also exhibits the angiocentric, angiodestructive pattern with infiltration of the brain parenchyma and leptomeninges by pleomorphic lymphoid and plasmacytoid cells (Fig. 7–5).

Characteristically, lymphomatoid granulomatosis does not involve the lymph nodes, spleen, or bone marrow. Involvement of the reticuloendothelial system suggests the possibility of a neoplastic transformation. Progression to lymphoreticular neoplasm, most com-

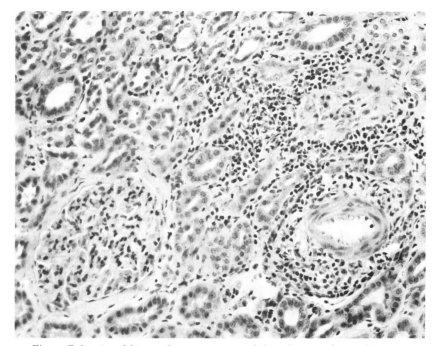

Figure 7–3. Renal biopsy from a patient with lymphomatoid granulomatosis. An interstitial and perivascular mononuclear cell infiltrate is present. Note that the adjacent glomerulus is normal in appearance. Hematoxylin and eosin stain (original magnification ×220).

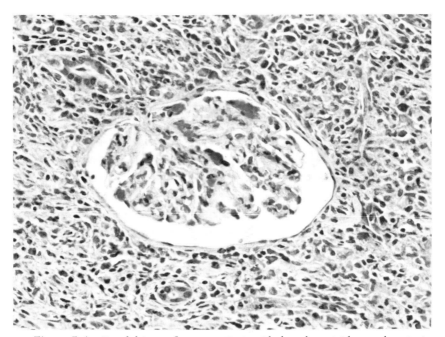

Figure 7–4. Renal biopsy from a patient with lymphomatoid granulomatosis. The extensive atypical mononuclear cell infiltrate surrounds a relatively normal-appearing glomerulus. Hematoxylin and eosin stain (original magnification ×330).

monly a non-Hodgkin's lymphoma, has been reported to occur in over 10 per cent of patients diagnosed as having lymphomatoid granulomatosis in a retrospective study.[379] However, in our prospective experience, this incidence has been closer to 50 per cent.

Skin lesions are frequently biopsied, and the angiodestructive pattern with pleomorphic mononuclear cells may be identified. Fat necrosis secondary to destructive vascular lesions may result in a predominant pattern of panniculitis on the biopsy specimen.

Diagnosis and differential diagnosis. The diagnosis of lymphomatoid granulomatosis is established by the finding of a pleomorphic mononuclear cell infiltrate around and within vessels, most commonly in a lung biopsy or skin biopsy. Because of the destructive nature of the infiltrate, an elastin stain may be required to demonstrate the vascular nature of the inflammatory process.

Figure 7–5. A, Brain biopsy from a patient with lymphomatoid granulomatosis. A rather homogeneous infiltrate of mononuclear cells surrounds the vein. Hematoxylin and eosin stain (original stain ×130). B, A more detailed view of the biopsy seen in A. Note the extension of the mononuclear cell infiltrate into the brain parenchyma. Hematoxylin and eosin stain (original magnification ×330).

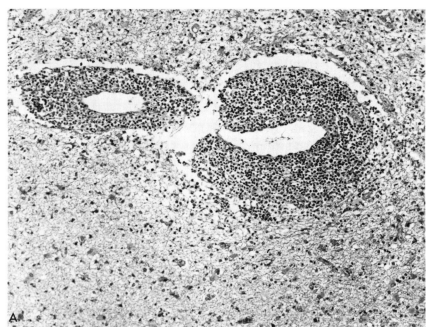

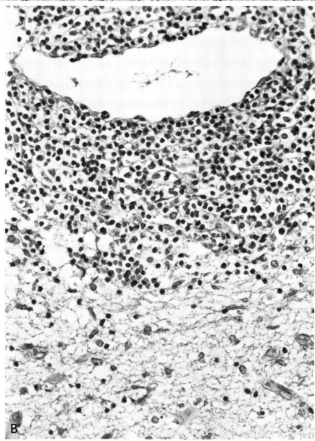

Figure 7–5. *See legend on opposite page.*

The differential diagnosis of lymphomatoid granulomatosis includes Wegener's granulomatosis including the limited form, pulmonary lymphoma, allergic angiitis and granulomatosis, lymphocytic interstitial pneumonia, and infectious granuloma.[388]

Major upper respiratory involvement, marked elevation of the ESR, and a glomerulonephritis suggest the diagnosis of Wegener's granulomatosis. The absence of glomerular involvement does not exclude the diagnosis of the limited form of Wegener's granulomatosis. A patient with granulomatous vasculitis and (1) pulmonary involvement without upper respiratory tract disease, (2) CNS or cutaneous disease or both, and (3) a normal white cell count and ESR is more likely to have lymphomatoid granulomatosis than Wegener's granulomatosis. A close evaluation of the histologic pattern may be required to make the distinction between these two diseases. A pleomorphic mononuclear infiltrate with relatively frequent mitotic figures favors the diagnosis of lymphomatoid granulomatosis, whereas the presence of increased numbers of polymorphonuclear cells and well-formed granulomata suggests the diagnosis of Wegener's granulomatosis.

Differentiation between a lymphoreticular neoplasm and lymphomatoid granulomatosis may be difficult. The absence of spleen, bone marrow, and hilar lymph node involvement favors the diagnosis of lymphomatoid granulomatosis. Major involvement of the reticuloendothelial system or a peripheral blood lymphocytosis suggests a lymphoreticular tumor or progression of the lymphomatoid granulomatosis to a neoplastic process. Because of the difficulty in differentiating between these two diagnostic possibilities, a complete systemic work-up similar to a staging evaluation is suggested, including an evaluation of the retroperitoneal space and bilateral bone marrow biopsies.

Allergic angiitis and granulomatosis may present with a similar clinical picture, but marked infiltration by eosinophils seen in allergic angiitis and granulomatosis is unusual in lymphomatoid granulomatosis. The frequent bowel and cardiac involvement also seen in allergic angiitis and granulomatosis is characteristically not seen in lymphomatoid granulomatosis.

The other diagnostic possibilities, including interstitial pneumonia and infectious causes of granuloma formation, do not normally involve pulmonary vessels. Special stains and appropriate cultures can help exclude infectious agents. Evidence of infectious agents may be present with lymphomatoid granulomatosis, however; for example, cytomegalic inclusions were demonstrated in the lung of 6 of 22 patients evaluated at autopsy.[11] These data remain to be confirmed, however.

Prognosis and treatment. It is extremely difficult to evaluate the mortality statistics for each of the phases of lymphomatoid granulomatosis since most, if not all, reports fail to take into account the different stages within the spectrum. It has been advocated that "benign lymphocytic angiitis and granulomatosis" not be treated.[95] However, follow-up studies have shown that untreated patients with disease at this stage can clearly progress to true lymphomatoid granulomatosis as well as go on to frank lymphoma.[374] We have aggressively treated patients who present with "benign lymphocytic angiitis and granulomatosis" with cyclophosphamide in the 2 mg per kg per day regimen together with alternate-day corticosteroids used for Wegener's granulomatosis and severe systemic necrotizing vasculitis and have noted striking remissions that have now been observed for years. Patients who initially present with lymphomatoid granulomatosis involving multiple organ systems have also been treated with this regimen. However, the prognosis in this group has been strikingly less favorable than that in the former group, with less than 50 per cent of patients attaining remission. Most of the patients who succumbed did so after transformation of their disease into an obvious neoplastic process. The therapy was not responsible for this, since untreated patients also developed neoplastic transformation. Both patients who present with lymphomatoid granulomatosis together with true lymphoproliferative disease as well as those who are observed to clearly progress from lymphomatoid granulomatosis to lymphoma have a uniformly poor prognosis despite various regimens of combined chemotherapy. However, it should be pointed out that these patients are usually treated aggressively with lymphoma-type chemotherapy regimens only late in the course of their disease.

The mortality statistics for this disease as they appear in the literature reflect the extremely poor prognosis of the disease as a whole,[379] taking into account that the various phases are grouped together. Over 90 per cent of the deaths occurred within 3 years, with a mean survival of just over 11 months. A similarly bleak prognosis has been reported by Israel et al.,[95] with eight of nine patients dying. Marked neurologic involvement, increased numbers of atypical cells in the inflammatory infiltrate, and progression to a frankly neoplastic process are poor prognostic signs.

Initial reports on therapeutic response in lymphomatoid granulomatosis have been generally negative. Prednisone as a single agent has been reported to produce transient improvement in the patient's clinical status, but recurrence of the disease is standard.[11] Israel et al.[95] reported a negative experience with prednisone in combination with various cytotoxic agents. Attempts at aggressive therapy of the CNS disease, including radiotherapy and intrathecal methotrexate, have not produced long-term remissions.[389] Radiotherapy alone may palliate local disease, but progression of disease at other sites is characteristic.[390]

As mentioned earlier, in contrast to this negative experience, a preliminary report suggests that some patients with lymphomatoid granulomatosis can be put into remission with the same combination of prednisone and cyclophosphamide utilized in patients with Wegener's granulomatosis.[374] Long-term remissions in patients with lymphomatoid granulomatosis can sometimes be achieved with this combination of cyclophosphamide and prednisone (Fauci AS, unpublished observation). Better results are obtained in patients who are treated early before widespread extensive disease involvement is present. Currently, we consider the prednisone-cyclophosphamide combination the treatment of choice for lymphomatoid granulomatosis prior to its transformation into a lymphoproliferative process.

CHAPTER 8

GIANT CELL ARTERITIDES

INTRODUCTION

The giant cell arteritides consist of two generally, but not invariably, distinct clinical syndromes, temporal arteritis and Takayasu's arteritis, which have in common a granulomatous vasculitis of medium- and large-sized arteries.

TEMPORAL ARTERITIS

Definition.   Temporal arteritis is a systemic panarteritis affecting predominantly elderly patients.[1, 391] Although any medium- or large-sized artery may be involved, the majority of clinical signs and symptoms result from vasculitis in branches of the carotid artery. The terms "cranial arteritis" or "giant arteritis" used to described this syndrome emphasize that the disease is not localized to the temporal arteries.

Historical perspective.   Hutchinson[12] in 1890 reported the first clinical description of temporal arteritis. In 1932 Horton et al.[14] recognized the presence of a granulomatous arteritis in this disease and subsequently further defined the clinical syndrome.[392] By 1938 Jennings[393] had recognized blindness as a complication of temporal arteritis. Gilmour[394] recognized the systemic nature of the disease process in 1941. In 1960 Paulley and Hughes[395] proposed a possible association between polymyalgia rheumatica (PMR) and the temporal arteritis syndrome.

Incidence and prevalence.   The overall incidence of this disease is 2.9 per 100,000 population per year.[396] The incidence per year per 100,000 population over 50 years of age increased from 5.1 in the 1950s to 17.4 in the 1970s.[397] This latter finding may well reflect a greater awareness of the disease with more thorough reporting. The age-specific incidence rate increased with age, rising from 1.7 in 50- to 59-year-old patients to 55.5 for patients over 80 years of age.[396] The overall prevalence is 24 cases per 100,000 population,[396] but it is 133 per 100,000 population aged 50 years and older.[397] Again, the prevalence increases with age and is 843 per 100,000 population aged 80 years and over.[396] Although in most large series[398, 399] greater than 95 per cent of patients are older than 50 years of age, several cases of biopsy-proven temporal arteritis have been reported in young adults and adolescents.[400, 401] There is a slight female predominance,[391, 398] and the average age at onset of symptoms is approximately 70 years.[398]

Pathophysiology. The etiology of this disease is unknown. The potential mechanisms for the expression of granulomatous vasculitis have been discussed in detail in Chapter 2. A substantial amount of indirect evidence points to an immune-mediated abnormality.[402-407] An association between hepatitis B infection and temporal arteritis has been suggested[402] but not found by all investigators.[403] Elevated serum IgG and complement levels are reported.[404] Using immunofluorescence, Liang et al.[405] demonstrated immunoglobulin in the temporal artery biopsies of patients with active disease, but the nature of the immunoglobulin was not further characterized. Waaler et al.[406] demonstrated anti-IgG rheumatoid factor–like activity (anti-Fc activity) in temporal artery biopsies with histologic evidence of active disease. This activity appeared to be mediated by IgA alone or in combination with IgG and IgM. The role of immune complexes in temporal arteritis requires further definition. An increased lymphocyte proliferative response to arterial antigen in patients with polymyalgia rheumatica has been suggested[407] but not demonstrated by all groups.[408] The significance of this observation with regard to the pathogenesis of temporal arteritis is unclear.

A possible role for environmental and genetic factors has been suggested.[391, 409, 410] The largest reported series of this disease comes from centers in more northern latitudes (reviewed in references 391 and 409) in the United States and Europe. Although well-documented cases have been reported, the disease seems to be rare in black Americans.[411-413] Familial aggregations of temporal arteritis and PMR have been reported.[409] An increased incidence of HLA-B8 tissue type[410] has been suggested in patients with temporal arteritis, but this relationship has not yet been confirmed by others.[403] These observations suggest that environmental and genetic factors may be important in the pathogenesis of this disease.

Clinical considerations. The initial symptoms of temporal arteritis are nonspecific (Table 8–1).[391, 398, 399, 414] In one series[398] the most common symptoms were headache (44 per cent), malaise (20 per cent), fatigue (12 per cent), and jaw claudication (12 per cent). With

TABLE 8–1.   INITIAL SYMPTOMS IN PATIENTS WITH
TEMPORAL ARTERITIS*

SYMPTOM	PERCENTAGE
Headache	44
Malaise	20
Fatigue	12
Jaw claudication	12
Extremity claudication	8
Fever	8
Arthralgias	8
Congestive heart failure	8
Tender scalp nodules	8

*The table summarizes the initial symptoms in 25 patients with biopsy-proven temporal arteritis reported in reference 398.

the exception of jaw claudication, these symptoms are nondiagnostic. Because of the nonspecific presentation, delays of up to 6 months from the onset of symptoms to an established diagnosis are common.

The signs and symptoms in patients with temporal arteritis are summarized in Table 8–2. The syndrome is noteworthy for its high incidence of nonspecific constitutional symptoms of fever, weight loss, anorexia, malaise, and depression. Rarely, the disease may present as a fever of unknown origin.[415]

HEADACHE.   Classically, the headache of temporal arteritis produces a continuous pain with a boring quality and intermittent lancinating exacerbations.[398] This pattern, however, is not uniformly present. Radiation of pain to the neck, face, jaws, or tongue may occur. The pain may worsen at night or with exposure to cold.

SYMPTOMS RELATED TO THE TEMPORAL ARTERY.   Abnormalities including tenderness, absent pulse, and nodules along the course of the temporal artery can be demonstrated in nearly one half the cases (Table 8–2). Unfortunately, these findings tend to appear later in the course of the disease and, consequently, are of less use in initially suggesting the diagnosis.[397-399, 412, 414, 416] Moreover, there is often a discrepancy between the physical findings and an abnormal temporal artery biopsy. In patients with the characteristic biopsy finding, approximately one third show no abnormal physical findings in the region of the temporal artery.[415, 417] Less common physical findings include hair loss, erythema, and necrosis along the path of the temporal artery.[418, 419]

OPHTHALMIC PROBLEMS.   Functional visual impairment occurs in 36 per cent of patients with temporal arteritis (Table 8–2). Although certain patients may present initially with sudden blindness without any previous symptoms, this is distinctly unusual.[398, 399] Most patients have definite symptoms of arteritis prior to onset of visual loss.[393, 399, 420] The mean time of symptoms prior to blindness is 3½

TABLE 8–2. SIGNS AND SYMPTOMS IN PATIENTS WITH
TEMPORAL ARTERITIS°

Sign or Symptom	Percentage†	Total Number of Patients
Constitutional		
Headache	60	729
Fever	48	421
Polymyalgia rheumatica‡	47	562
Weight loss	45	339
Anorexia	36	154
Malaise	29	160
Depression	25	211
Specific		
Localized to artery		
Tenderness	55	296
Absent pulse	51	138
Nodules	35	150
Ophthalmic		
Visual impairment	36	819
Blindness (sustained)	16	146
Amaurosis fugax	12	437
Diplopia	12	472
Claudication		
Jaw	36	424
Extremity	8	196
Other		
Facial neuralgia	21	183
Vertigo	12	172

°Data are summarized from a literature review compiled by Goodman.[391]
†Percentage of total number of patients for whom a given sign or symptom was positive.
‡Includes symptoms of arthralgia, myalgias, and stiffness.

months. Unfortunately, the majority of these symptoms are nonspecific and diagnosis may not be made prior to the decrease in vision.[398] Physical examination of the eye usually is not helpful in evaluating the risk of blindness. In the majority of cases, the visual loss results from an ischemic optic neuritis, and the funduscopic examination may be normal for 1 to 2 days after the onset of blindness.[420] Less frequently, decreased visual acuity is caused by central retinal artery occlusion or retrobulbar involvement. Orbital bruits, if present, may suggest an increased risk of ocular involvement.[421]

Diplopia occurs in 12 per cent of cases. The transient ophthalmoplegia may result either from ischemia of cranial nerves III, IV, or VI or from ischemia of the extraocular muscles.[422, 423] Although ophthalmoplegia is a relatively rare symptom, it is clinically important. Diplopia preceded the onset of blindness in over 50 per cent of patients.[399, 424] The loss of vision in one eye also appears to increase the risk of visual impairment in the remaining eye.[399]

CLAUDICATION. Unlike the majority of nonspecific symptoms, jaw claudication, which is present in one third of patients, is characteristic of temporal arteritis. Pain is brought on by mastication or talking and is relieved by rest. Of interest is the fact that bruits were heard over the large systemic arteries in the majority of patients in one series[425]; in spite of this observation, claudication of other sites such as extremities, tongue, or pharyngeal muscles is uncommon. Progression to ischemic infarction, arterial aneurysm formation, and arterial wall dissection appears to be quite rare.

Unusual findings in this disease have been recently summarized and include vertigo, hearing loss, sore throat, epistaxis, glossitis, blanching tongue, carpal tunnel syndrome, and visual hallucination.[391]

POLYMYALGIA RHEUMATICA. PMR is a clinical syndrome of unknown etiology seen most commonly in individuals over the age of 50 years. It is characterized by proximal muscle pain, periarticular pain, and morning stiffness.[426, 427] Constitutional symptoms such as malaise, weight loss, and fever are also common. The relationship between PMR and temporal arteritis suggested by Paulley and Hughes is now firmly established.[428-432] Patients with temporal arteritis have a symptom complex consistent with PMR in 47 per cent of cases (Table 8–2), and from 40 to 50 per cent of patients with PMR have positive temporal artery biopsies in the absence of specific symptoms related to the head.[432, 433] With this degree of overlap, it is difficult to make a clinical distinction between these two disease entities. Eye involvement may develop in patients with the PMR syndrome.[428] Moreover, low-dose corticosteroid treatment may suppress the symptom complex of PMR but be inadequate to prevent ocular disease.

Laboratory consideration. The common laboratory findings in temporal arteritis include a mild normochromic, normocytic anemia that is refractory to replacement therapy. An abnormal erythrocyte sedimentation rate (ESR) with marked elevations is characteristic,[391] although cases with normal values have been reported.[434] The presence of anemia and an elevated ESR in an elderly patient with nonspecific symptoms should suggest the diagnosis of temporal arteritis.[435] Other laboratory parameters include normal to elevated IgG and complement levels and elevated acute-phase reactants such as α_2 globulin and fibrinogen.

The frequency of abnormal liver function studies has also been emphasized.[436-439] The most common finding is an elevated alkaline phosphatase although, less frequently, a mild elevation of hepatic transaminases has been noted. A liver biopsy in a case of PMR with hepatic involvement showed a granulomatous hepatitis rather than a vasculitis.[438]

Pathology. Pathologic findings in temporal arteritis have been

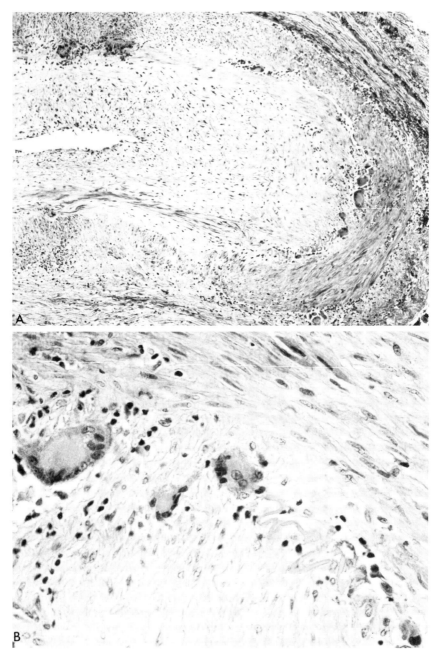

Figure 8–1. A, Temporal artery biopsy from a patient with temporal arteritis. A mononuclear cell infiltrate and several multinucleated giant cells are seen. Note the extensive endothelial cell proliferation and narrowing of the vascular lumen. Hematoxylin and eosin stain (original magnification ×80). B, A detailed view of the temporal artery biopsy seen in A. A cluster of multinucleated giant cells is seen adjacent to a disrupted elastic membrane. Hematoxylin and eosin stain (original magnification × 330).

studies in detail.[431] The disease is characterized by a panarteritis with an inflammatory reaction consisting of mononuclear cells, polymorphonuclear leukocytes, and eosinophils (Fig. 8–1). Veins and smaller vessels are spared. The major site of involvement is the media, with smooth muscle necrosis and interruption of the internal elastic membrane. Giant cells are present to varying degrees and may be quite rare.[395, 425] The degree of intimal proliferation is also variable and may progress to occlusion of the vessels. The segmental nature of the inflammation in temporal arteritis has been emphasized repeatedly.[440, 441]

Although involvement of the superficial temporal arteries is widely recognized in this disease, vertebral, ophthalmic, and posterior ciliary artery involvement is also common.[442] Internal carotid, external carotid, and central retinal arteries are less frequently affected. Although cases of cerebral artery involvement are reported,[443] generally the intracranial circulation is spared.[442]

It should be emphasized that despite the nomenclature, temporal arteritis is a systemic disease, and its systemic nature with the potential for involvement of any intermediate- or large-sized muscular artery is now well established clinically and pathologically.[414, 425, 431, 444] Indeed, a clinical syndrome similar to polyarteritis nodosa (PAN) may on rare occasions be seen in patients with giant cell arteritis.[445] Involvement of arteries in muscles seems to be quite rare.[431] It is important to emphasize that despite the systemic nature of temporal arteritis, symptoms of ischemia or necrosis below the neck are not common.

Diagnosis and differential diagnosis. The diagnosis may be established by biopsy, most commonly of the temporal artery. Because of the segmental nature of the arteritis, care in handling the biopsy specimens has been emphasized. The use of superficial temporal angiography to define areas with abnormalities has been suggested.[446-448] Arteriography may aid in establishing an optimal biopsy site but is not of itself diagnostic.[448] Large or even bilateral biopsies of the temporal arteries with serial sections of the specimen have been proposed to increase the diagnostic yield.[440, 441]

It should also be noted that other systemic vasculitic processes, such as PAN, may involve the temporal artery (see Chapter 4). In this regard, evaluation of patients with temporal artery vasculitis with and without giant cells showed significant differences between the two groups.[449, 450] The latter group (patients without giant cells) had significantly increased mortality, with evidence of PAN found at autopsy in several cases. The distinction is potentially important clinically because corticosteroid therapy alone may be inadequate for certain types of systemic necrotizing vasculitis (see Chapter 4). If a temporal artery biopsy demonstrates a vasculitis in the absence of giant cells, a more extensive systemic evaluation for visceral vasculitis should be considered.

The differential diagnosis of temporal arteritis includes a wide variety and number of disease entities.[391] Each pattern of presentation may be associated with a different group of diseases in the differential diagnosis.

HEADACHE.   Other causes such as migraine headache, intracranial disease, and referred pain from problems in the facial structures should be excluded.

ARTHRALGIA-MYALGIA.   This nonspecific symptom complex may be seen in a wide variety of diseases ranging from mild viral syndromes to inflammatory processes, such as the connective tissue diseases, to occult malignancies. Symptoms persisting for longer than 1 month warrant a complete evaluation.

FACIAL PAIN.   Neuralgia, inflammatory or neoplatic diseases of the facial structures, temporomandibular joint dysfunction, and referred cardiac pain should be included in the differential diagnosis.

SYSTEMIC ILLNESS IN THE AGED.   In the elderly, symptoms of systemic diseases may be nondiagnostic. Fever, anorexia, malaise, and weight loss may accompany occult infections, undiagnosed neoplasms, and abnormalities of thyroid function.

Sudden Blindness.   The diagnosis of sudden blindness from optic neuritis, retrobulbar neuritis, or central retinal artery or vein occlusion in an elderly patient suggests the possibility of temporal arteritis. To establish the diagnosis, a high index of suspicion and knowledge of the many clinical manifestations are required.

Treatment and prognosis.   Most patients with temporal arteritis respond dramatically to corticosteroid therapy. Within days, systemic symptoms of fever, malaise, and musculoskeletal pain begin to resolve.[398] Focal manifestations of vascular disease, such as claudication, headache, or scalp tenderness, also resolve. The efficacy of corticosteroids in preventing blindness and other vascular complications is well established. For this reason, rapid establishment of diagnosis and initiation of appropriate therapy are highly desirable.

Treatment is started initially with 40 to 60 mg of prednisone orally per day. Upon control of the disease, the prednisone is tapered to a maintenance dose, generally in the range of 7.5 to 10 mg per day. Serial determinations of ESR may be helpful in monitoring steroid therapy. However, it should be pointed out that in the adjustment of corticosteroid dose regimens, particularly in tapering the dose after a patient has achieved remission, the ESR may rise slightly. If the patient remains symptom-free, the tapering can be cautiously continued, since recognizable symptoms almost invariably precede relapse with or without visual problems. The importance of prolonged therapy for 1 to 2 years has been emphasized.[451] The initial use of an alternate-day prednisone regimen is ineffective in controlling the symptoms of temporal arteritis.[452] Nonsteroidal anti-inflammatory agents are not effective in preventing the ocular complications.

With rapid diagnosis and appropriate treatment prior to a life-threatening ischemic event, the prognosis is excellent and the patient will have a normal life expectancy.[397] In general, visual impairment is not reversible, although functional vision is restored in a minority of cases.[453] Most patients will achieve complete remission and can eventually be tapered off the prednisone. Relapses do occur; consequently, follow-up evaluations are a necessity.

TAKAYASU'S ARTERITIS

Definition. Takayasu's arteritis is a disease characterized by inflammation and stenosis of large- and intermediate-sized arteries with frequent involvement of the aortic arch and its branches.[454-457] The disease most frequently affects young women, and its cause is unknown.

Historical perspective. Davy[458] in 1839 and Savory[459] in 1856 reported the first cases of Takayasu's arteritis. Takayasu[13] in 1908 drew attention to unusual changes in the retina of a young woman. In the discussion that followed Takayasu's presentation, Onishi and Kagoshima[13] made the association between the unusual retinal changes and absent radial pulses. Judge et al.[460] have reviewed in detail the historical evolution of the understanding of Takayasu's arteritis. A wide variety of names have been applied to this disease, including Martorell's syndrome, Raeder-Harbit's syndrome, aortic arch syndrome, aortic arch arteritis, brachial arteritis, reverse coarctation, obliterative arteritis of the carotid and subclavian arteries, pulseless disease, pulseless syndrome, chronic subclavio-carotid obstruction, and arteritis of the aorta in young women.

Pathophysiology. The etiology of Takayasu's arteritis is unknown. Several observations, however, are of interest. Evidence of infection with tuberculosis was reported in several series.[461, 462] A toxic effect from *Mycobacterium tuberculosis* has been suggested,[461] but no direct evidence supports this hypothesis. The relationship, if any, between tuberculosis and Takayasu's arteritis is at best uncertain. Evidence of a recent streptococcal infection was found in over half the patients in another series,[463] but this association was not seen in the majority of reports.

The possibility of an immune-mediated etiology has been proposed. The majority of patients have elevated immunoglobulins. Several reports suggest the presence of antibody directed against components of the artery,[464-466] but negative observations have also been reported.[467, 468] The significance of these observations with regard to the pathophysiology of Takayasu's arteritis is unclear. Genetic factors may be significant in this disease, and the female predominance is striking. In this regard, increased secretion of estrogen products in the urine has been reported in patients with Takayasu's arteritis.[469] However, the precise role of estrogen in this disease has not been defined. An increased incidence of HLA-B5,[470, 471] A10,[471] Bw52,[472] and HLA-DHO[473] has also been recorded. The disease has been seen in monozygotic twins.[474] These latter observations strongly suggest the importance of genetic factors. However, despite these reported observations, the etiology and precise pathophysiology of this disease are entirely unknown.

Incidence and prevalence. Takayasu's arteritis is a rare disease. Up until 1972, just over 300 cases had been reported.[455] There is a marked female predominance, with a ratio of almost 9 to 1. The disease affects young women, the majority of patients in most series presenting with the disease between the ages of 15 and 20 years. Although originally believed to be a disease of Oriental women, its worldwide distribution and racial heterogeneity are now well recognized.[475, 476]

Clinical considerations. Clinical manifestations of Takayasu's arteritis are summarized in Table 8–3. The disease has been divided into an acute stage, characterized by signs and symptoms of a systemic inflammatory process, followed by a chronic phase, characterized by signs and symptoms of vascular occlusion. A mean of 8 years with a range of months to decades between the two phases has been reported.[468] The frequency with which an acute inflammatory disease is identified prior to the occlusive stage varies markedly with different series, but a figure of 70 per cent has been suggested.[478] Obviously, a delay of years between the phases makes evaluation of this relationship difficult.

The acute inflammatory phase of Takayasu's arteritis was initially emphasized in reported series from Scandinavia[479, 480] and was subsequently reviewed.[468, 478] The presentation is a nonspecific pattern of a systemic inflammatory process. Fever, night sweats, malaise, weakness, myalgias, and arthralgias are characteristic. Arthritis with single- or multiple-joint involvement and a migratory pattern has been described. Episcleritis, iritis, and skin involvement with painful nodules are less frequent findings. Pulmonary involvement with pleuritic chest pain as well as hemoptysis has also been reported. Pericarditis and Raynaud's phenomenon are less frequently reported.

In contrast to the nonspecific symptoms of the acute stage of Takayasu's arteritis, the signs and symptoms associated with the chronic phase of the disease reflect ischemia of the involved organ system. Of note, symptoms of vascular insufficiency may be the presenting complaint.[476, 481, 482] Involvement by organ systems is summarized in Table 8–3. An unusual posture related to vascular insufficiency is described in patients with Takayasu's arteritis and is characterized by flexion of the neck with a "face-down" position.[481] Patients assume this posture to avoid transient decreases in visual

TABLE 8-3. CLINICAL MANIFESTATIONS OF
TAKAYASU'S ARTERITIS*

CLINICAL MANIFESTATION	PERCENTAGE†	TOTAL NUMBER OF PATIENTS
General		
"Face-down" posture	65	110
Fatigue/malaise	59	211
Headache	57	237
Fever	20	84
Weight loss	14	211
Organ System		
Vascular		
Absent pulses	98	217
Radial	100	110
Ulnar	76	20
Carotid	52	130
Axillary	15	20
Femoral	5	20
Sensitive carotid sinus	87	110
Bruits	86	175
Carotid	50	20
Supraclavicular	35	20
Abdominal	10	20
Femoral	0	20
Hypertension	59	236
Claudication	37	123
Pain over artery	32	84
Raynaud's phenomenon	10	20
Ocular		
Difficulty looking up	60	48
Hypertensive retinal changes	41	107
Retinal vessel anastomoses	33	217
Altered vision	26	189
Cataracts	15	217
Central Nervous System		
Syncope	51	217
Hemiplegia	7	189
Cardiac		
Dyspnea	48	194
Palpitations	43	194
Congestive heart failure	36	107
Left-sided	28	107
Right-sided	8	107
Angina	12	194
Pericarditis	3	107
Gastrointestinal Tract		
Nausea/vomiting	15	211

*Data are summarized from references 454–456, 465, 475, and 477.
†Percentage of total number of patients for whom a given clinical manifestation was positive.

acuity and narrowing of visual fields caused by an exacerbation of vascular insufficiency, which may occur with the head in the extended "face-up" position.

VASCULAR MANIFESTATIONS. Signs of vascular abnormalities are found in nearly all patients. Absence of at least one arterial pulse is recorded for 98 per cent of patients (Table 8–3). Radial, ulnar, and carotid arteries are the most frequently involved sites. Bruits can be found in 86 per cent of patients, the vast majority being identified in the neck of supraclavicular region. The bruit is present in systole and in some cases extends into diastole, reflecting flow through collaterals. Symptoms of arterial involvement such as claudication (37 per cent), pain over an artery (particularly the carotid artery) (32 per cent), and Raynaud's phenomenon are somewhat less frequent. The symptoms of claudication are found with equal frequency in the upper and lower extremities.[455]

HYPERTENSION. An elevation of blood pressure is present in over half the patients with Takayasu's arteritis (Table 8–3). The need to evaluate leg blood pressure readings has been emphasized[477] because of the potential for spuriously low readings in the arm. The elevation of blood pressure is multifactorial in origin. Important mechanisms include loss of vascular compliance due to the underlying disease and renal vascular ischemia.[462, 477] The role of decreased cerebral blood flow with increased sensitivity of the carotid sinus reflex in hypertension is uncertain and has been debated. In this regard, elevated peripheral blood renin levels were reported in the absence of renal artery involvement and were reduced by obliterations of the carotid sinus nerves.[483] This observation suggests that disease involvement of the carotid arteries as well as the renal arteries can produce hyperreninemia and contribute to the pathogenesis of hypertension. The importance of a given mechanism probably varies with each patient.

OCULAR MANIFESTATIONS. Difficulty in looking up is noted by 60 per cent of patients, resulting in the "face-down" posture previously mentioned. Transient visual impairment may result if the head is extended. The most common fundoscopic abnormalities are the changes secondary to hypertension. The retinal changes emphasized by Takayasu[13] are found in only one third of patients (Table 8–3). These changes, which are arteriovenous anastomoses, are caused by ischemia and are not local vasculitis. Cataracts and ischemic damage to the anterior structures of the eye are seen in a minority of patients.

CENTRAL NERVOUS SYSTEM. Over one half the patients have experienced syncopal episodes (Table 8–3). Paresthesias are also frequently described. Cerebral infarction is less frequent, with hemiplegia being present in 7 per cent of patients.

CARDIOPULMONARY MANIFESTATIONS. Palpitation and dyspnea are frequent complaints, and congestive heart failure is present in over one third of patients. Both left-sided and right-sided heart failure patterns are described and generally reflect systemic and pulmonary hypertension, respectively. Less frequently, aortic insufficiency secondary to aortitis or aortic valve involvement may contribute to the clinical picture.[457, 484] Rarely, myocarditis and pericarditis are noted.[485] Angina pectoris is seen in 12 per cent of patients. Although coronary artery ischemia may result from the increased preload, vasculitis of the proximal coronary arteries is a well-documented complication of this disease.[484, 486]

PREGNANCY. Because Takayasu's arteritis is a disease of young women, the effect of pregnancy on the disease assumes major importance. In a disease that can cause vascular compromise of the central nervous system, heart, kidney, lungs, and pelvis, the increased vascular stress of pregnancy could result in increased morbidity. However, normal pregnancy, labor, and delivery have been reported in patients with Takayasu's arteritis[455, 487, 488]; approximately one half the patients will have exacerbations and one half will experience improvements in the symptoms of their disease during pregnancy.[482] Cesarean sections are reserved for purely obstetric indications.[488]

Cause of death. In two large clinical series,[454, 456] 7 and 14 per cent of patients died, respectively. The most common cause of death was congestive heart failure followed by myocardial infarction and sudden unexplained death. Less frequently, renal failure and intracranial bleeding were the cause of death.

Laboratory. Routine blood studies may show a mild anemia or mild leukocytosis, or may be entirely normal. The ESR is elevated in the great majority of patients. Immunoglobulins IgG, IgA, and IgM tend to be elevated, while rheumatoid factor and antinuclear antibodies are generally negative.[489]

X-ray studies are important in the evaluation of Takayasu's arteritis. Suggestive findings can be seen on routine chest radiographs and include widening of the aortic shadow, irregularities of the descending aorta, aortic calcification, pulmonary arterial changes, cardiac enlargement, hilar fullness or masses, and rib-notching from collaterals.[456, 490] Pleural effusions have been reported but appear to be unusual.[491]

The important role of arteriography in the diagnosis and evaluation of Takayasu's arteritis has been emphasized.[454-456, 492] Arteriographic findings include narrowing to complete occlusion of large arteries with collateral circulation (Fig. 8–2). Aneurysms, including both saccular and fusiform patterns, are often present. The frequency of vessel involvement by anatomic site is summarized in Table 8–4. The most commonly involved sites are the subclavian artery, descending aorta, renal artery, and carotid artery. The more frequent involvement of the pulmonary artery, which approaches 50 per cent, has recently been emphasized.[457]

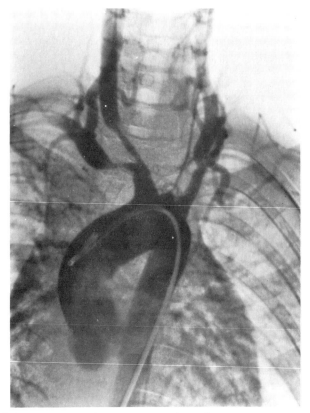

Figure 8-2. An aortic arch angiogram with a subtraction view in a woman with Takayasu's arteritis. Diffuse vessel disease with particularly severe involvement of the proximal right subclavian and carotid arteries is seen.

TABLE 8-4. *ARTERIAL INVOLVEMENT IN TAKAYASU'S ARTERITIS AS DETERMINED BY ANGIOGRAPHY***

ARTERY	PERCENTAGE†	TOTAL NUMBER OF PATIENTS
Subclavian	83	127
Descending aorta	58	127
Renal	56	127
Carotid	43	127
Ascending aorta	30	127
Abdominal aorta	20	20
Vertebral	19	127
Iliac	17	127
Innominate	16	127
Pulmonary	15	107
Mesenteric	15	107
Coronary	9	107
Femoral	8	127
Brachial	6	127

*Data are summarized from references 455 and 456.
†Percentage of total number of patients for whom a given site was involved.

Noninvasive studies may also be useful in follow-up evaluation. Echocardiography can be used to evaluate the aortic root.[493] Two-dimensional echocardiograms can be used to distinguish between aortic root dilatation and enlargement from a dissecting aneurysm. Other noninvasive tests to measure blood flow, such as Doppler flow studies and ophthalmodynamometry, can be used for serial follow-up evaluation.

Pathology. Takayasu's arteritis is characterized by a panarteritis of large elastic arteries with infiltration of all layers of the arterial wall with mononuclear cells and giant cells.[475, 494] Additional findings include intimal proliferation, fibrosis, disruption of the elastic lamina, and vascularization of the media (Fig. 8–3). Aneurysms of varying sizes can be seen,[494] but dissection and hemorrhage are much less frequent. The disease may be restricted to the aortic arch or its branches, involve thoracic and abdominal vessels, or diffusely involve the aorta and branches throughout the chest and abdominal cavities.[454] Pulmonary artery involvement is well documented.[457] Vessels initially damaged by the inflammatory process often manifest secondary atherosclerotic changes. Changes secondary to ischemia or hypertension are frequently noted. Tissue infarction is less common when the occlusive process is slow, allowing for development of collateral circulation.

Diagnosis and differential diagnosis. The diagnosis is generally established by the finding of characteristic changes on angiographic studies. Less frequently, tissue obtained during surgery from an appropriate vessel will have the characteristic findings.

The diagnosis of Takayasu's arteritis should be considered when symptoms of vascular insufficiency, such as pulse deficits, discrepancy in blood pressure determinations, vascular bruits, syncope, transient alterations in vision, claudication, or angina, are present in a young woman. The presence of a painful artery is also highly suggestive.

There are a few clinical syndromes that can be confused with Takayasu's arteritis. Several disease entities are associated with an aortitis and should be excluded.[495] Syphilitic aortitis, mycotic aneurysms, and aortitis secondary to rheumatic fever can be excluded by appropriate culture and serologic studies. X-ray studies of the spine and sacroiliac joints will exclude ankylosing spondylitis. The classic clinical presentations in relapsing polychondritis and Reiter's syndrome will help to rule out these diagnostic possibilities.

Treatment and prognosis. Corticosteroids are generally, but not uniformly, effective in suppressing the initial inflammatory symptoms of the disease.[454] However, the efficacy of corticosteroids in prolonging life is not well established. Recent studies suggest that prednisone, 30 mg per day, followed by chronic maintenance therapy in the range of 5 to 10 mg per day will prevent the long-term vascular complications and improve survival.[455, 457] Long-term follow-up will be

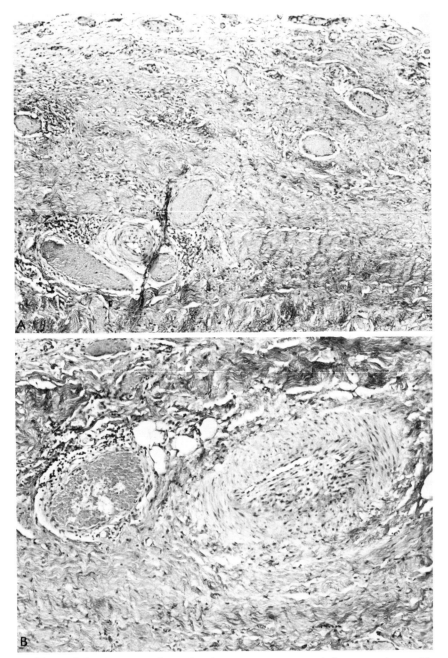

Figure 8-3. A, Tissue from the thoracic aorta removed from a patient with Takayasu's arteritis during a vascular bypass grafting procedure. Diffuse mononuclear cell infiltrate and neovascularization of the thickened aortic wall are seen. Hematoxylin and eosin (original magnification ×80). B, A detailed view of the aortic tissue shown in A. A large vasa vasorum with near-occlusion of its lumen is seen. Note the perivascular cuffing around the adjacent vein. Hematoxylin and eosin stain (original magnification ×100).

required to confirm these preliminary observations. The role of cytotoxic therapy in this disease has not yet been evaluated.

Vascular surgery can be useful in treating selected patients.[486, 496-498] Reconstructive surgery should be avoided during periods of active inflammatory disease, if possible. Avoidance of prosthetic materials has been suggested,[496, 497] but successful use of prosthetic grafts has been reported.[498] Generally, the experience of renal artery reconstruction has been negative,[496] but successful coronary artery bypass grafting has been reported.[486]

General medical management considerations are important in this group of patients. Hypertension is a major contributory factor in the evolution of congestive heart failure in patients with Takayasu's arteritis. Management of blood pressure may help to prevent some of the long-term sequelae. Obviously, care should be taken to avoid hypotension in this clinical setting. The finding of elevated peripheral renins[483] in this disease suggests that renin antagonists may be effective. Clinical experience, however, is currently lacking. Atherosclerosis may also play a contributory role in the late vascular events in Takayasu's arteritis. In this regard, evaluation of the blood lipid profile seems prudent. Finally, avoidance of drugs, such as estrogen or ergot compounds, with the potential to cause vascular complications also seems reasonable.

CHAPTER 9

VASCULITIS AND NEOPLASM

INTRODUCTION

Several clinical syndromes in which a vasculitic disease is associated with a neoplasm have been described. These syndromes are rare and are generally reported as separate cases in small series. In the present chapter these neoplasm-associated vasculitic syndromes are grouped by the pattern of the vasculitis and discussed under the following headings: (1) Systemic Necrotizing Vasculitis, (2) Granulomatous Vasculitis, (3) Hypersensitivity Vasculitis, and (4) Other Systemic Vasculitides Associated with Neoplasms. Following the discussion of the clinical syndromes, pathophysiologic considerations are reviewed. Finally, the vasculopathy associated with an atrial myxoma is discussed.

SYSTEMIC NECROTIZING VASCULITIS

Hairy cell leukemia and classic polyarteritis nodosa (PAN). Hairy cell leukemia is a distinctive form of chronic leukemia characterized by pancytopenia, splenomegaly in the absence of adenopathy, and circulating mononuclear cells with prominent cytoplasmic projections.[499, 500] Although the origin of the hairy cell is debated, most studies indicate that it is of B cell or monocyte lineage.[501]

The association between hairy cell leukemia and PAN was suggested by Elkon and colleagues when 4 of 138 patients with this unusual chronic leukemia developed vasculitis.[128, 502] The diagnosis of hairy cell leukemia predated the clinical manifestations of vasculitis by 6 months to a year in three of the four cases. The clinical course of this group of patients did not differ from the clinical course of patients with hairy cell leukemia as a whole except for the presence of

116

polyarthritis in one individual. It is of interest that PAN developed within 1 year of splenectomy in three of the four patients.

The manifestations of vasculitis in the patients with hairy cell leukemia were similar to those in patients with PAN without leukemia. Acute and chronic inflammation of medium-sized muscular arteries was present, and the characteristic pattern of aneurysm formation was found in angiographic studies. Peripheral artery aneurysms and temporal artery involvement were present in two of the four patients. We have also seen temporal artery involvement and peripheral aneurysms in a patient with hairy cell leukemia and PAN, a finding that is most unusual in patients with classic PAN.

Laboratory findings were remarkable for leukopenia and circulating hairy cells, which are characteristic for this chronic leukemia. In one patient studied, low complement levels and circulating immune complexes were demonstrated.

Given the small number of patients, it is difficult to evaluate the effect of therapy. Both corticosteroids and cyclophosphamide have been used.[128] A major problem in using cytotoxic agents in this group is the presence of pancytopenia, which increases the risk of leukopenia during therapy. In addition, patients with hairy cell leukemia are more prone to infections,[499, 500] reflecting, in part, decreased numbers and depressed functional capabilities of polymorphonuclear leukocytes and monocytes. Very close monitoring of the white blood cell count is obviously required in this subset of patients. Therapy for the underlying leukemia at present is only palliative. The outlook for these patients will, at best, reflect the prognosis of the underlying leukemia. In this regard, it should be pointed out that in a single patient under our care with hairy cell leukemia and systemic necrotizing vasculitis of the classic PAN type, cyclophosphamide and prednisone therapy resulted in a complete remission of the PAN, while the leukemia relentlessly progressed, leading to the death of the patient (Goedert et al., unpublished observations).

Malignant melanoma and allergic angiitis and granulomatosis. Recently, we evaluated a 31-year-old woman with a history of asthma since 1971. In 1974 the patient had an excisional biopsy of a malignant melanoma, but no evidence of metastatic disease was present. The patient's subsequent course was complicated by recurrent episodes of wheezing, pulmonary infiltrates, and peripheral eosinophilia. The bronchospasm and infiltrates were responsive initially to prednisone. After developing cardiomegaly and congestive heart failure, the patient was transferred to the NIH for evaluation in May 1979. Following a complete evaluation, a systemic necrotizing vasculitis with granuloma and eosinophilic infiltrates was demonstrated in lung, colon, and skin biopsies, confirming the diagnosis of allergic angiitis and granulomatosis. The patient had a dramatic response to prednisone and cyclophosphamide therapy. Five months later, skin nodules showed recurrent malignant melanoma and the patient subsequently died of a widely disseminated tumor.

The patient's case is unique. The temporal association of systemic necrotizing vasculitis and malignant melanoma raises the possibility of a relationship between the two disease processes. If there is an association between solid tumors and systemic necrotizing vasculitis, it is relatively rare. In this case, the vasculitis was well controlled, but the malignant melanoma progressed to a rapidly fatal outcome.

GRANULOMATOUS VASCULITIS

Hodgkin's disease and central nervous system (CNS) granulomatous angiitis. The quite rare association between lymphoma and CNS granulomatous angiitis is established by at least five well-documented cases.[503-508] In one series, only 1 of 18 patients with granulomatous angiitis had Hodgkin's disease.[509] In contrast, in a report of diseases associated with over 1000 patients with Hodgkin's disease, two cases of PAN were noted but no isolated CNS vasculitis was found.[510]

The clinical presentation of this group of patients is of particular interest. In two patients, symptoms related to CNS dysfunction were present more than 18 months before the diagnosis of lymphoma was established. In two patients, the CNS symptoms coincided with a course of radiotherapy to the chest, and in the fifth patient onset of symptoms related to cerebral arteritis followed 3 years of chemotherapy for the lymphoma.

The CNS dysfunction consisted of symptom complexes that suggested multifocal involvement. Altered mental status with deteriorating higher cortical function, seizure activity, and motor and sensory abnormalities was commonly reported. In two patients an abrupt deterioration of the CNS problems closely followed the initiation of cranial radiotherapy. The presence of disseminated herpes zoster seen in four of the five patients at the time of presentation of the CNS angiitis was emphasized.[505, 506] The varicella-zoster virus had been suggested as an etiologic agent of the vasculitis, but attempts to demonstrate viral particles in brain biopsy tissue from one patient were unsuccessful.[505]

Laboratory studies are relatively nondiagnostic. Cerebrospinal fluids showed initially elevated proteins, which tended to increase in serial studies. A mild pleocytosis consisting of mononuclear cells was the most common pattern. Cerebral angiography was the only test that seemed useful in establishing a premorbid diagnosis. Patterns of shifted anterior cerebral arteries,[504, 506] multiple aneurysms,[508] and occlusions of multiple vessels[506] were described.

Autopsy findings are available for three patients. Arteries of the leptomeninges and those perforating the brain tissue were the most commonly involved vessels, with relative sparing of the larger intracranial vessels. Involvement of the spinal cord was also noted. The histologic picture was a panarteritis with infiltrations by mononuclear cells including lymphocytes, monocytes, and "histiocyte-like" cells. Multinucleated giant cells were present in varying numbers. The vascular elastic membrane was either disrupted or, in some cases, left intact. Of note, all three patients dying with active cerebral vasculitis had residual or recurrent lymphoma. However, no neoplastic cells could be identified in the CNS.

In one of two patients with this syndrome who survived, treatment for the underlying Hodgkin's disease with radiotherapy to the chest was temporally associated with improvement in the CNS-related symptoms. One week after radiation therapy was started, dexamethasone was added to the regimen and 1 month later cyclic chemotherapy with MOPP (nitrogen mustard, vincristine, procarbazine, prednisone) was started, with continued improvement of CNS symptoms.

In the second patient who survived with this syndrome, evidence of neurologic dysfunction was noted several months after completion of a course of total nodal radiotherapy during a varicella-zoster infection of the trigeminal nerve.[508] The patient was diagnosed as having varicella-zoster encephalitis. No additional therapy was started, and the patient recovered. Two months later the patient developed weakness of the left arm. Eventually, a cerebral angiogram was performed, which showed multiple areas of narrowing and dilatation. No therapy was started and the patient subsequently developed an intracerebral bleeding diagnosed by computer-assisted tomographic scan. The patient survived this episode, but no long-term follow-up or status of the Hodgkin's disease was reported.

The following treatment approach, although based on only two case reports, would seem prudent until further information is available. If the therapy for Hodgkin's disease includes chemotherapy (i.e., MOPP), it may be effective in controlling the arteritis also. If the tumor treatment is limited to radiation therapy, additional immunosuppressive therapy for the angiitis may be indicated.

HYPERSENSITIVITY VASCULITIS

A pattern of hypersensitivity vasculitis can be seen with a variety of neoplastic diseases, including Hodgkin's disease, other lymphomas, multiple myeloma, and carcinoma.[239, 316, 511] Although significant numbers of patients with hypersensitivity vasculitis have been reported to have an underlying neoplasm,[315, 511] in our experience neoplasm is a relatively rare underlying cause of hypersensitivity vasculitis. It is important to note that cutaneous vasculitis may precede the clinical presentation of the tumor by weeks to years. There are few data on the response of the vasculitis to therapy. Corticosteroid therapy has not been particularly helpful.[316] Improvements, however, have been observed when the underlying neoplastic process is controlled.

OTHER SYSTEMIC VASCULITIDES ASSOCIATED WITH NEOPLASMS

The association of Raynaud's phenomenon with carcinoma and lymphoreticular tumors has been suggested.[512, 513] Progression to ischemic infarction and gangrene was observed in some of the reported cases. Friedman and colleagues[514] presented angiographic and histologic evidence that a vasculitic process causes this syndrome in at least some patients. Tissue from a digital artery in a patient with an epidermoid carcinoma of the cervix demonstrated infiltration by lymphocytes and polymorphonuclear leukocytes, necrosis, and intimal proliferation. In the majority of patients the picture of extremity ischemia was present from weeks to months before the diagnosis of cancer was established. The symptoms related to the angiitis appeared to stabilize if the neoplastic process was controlled.

Mononeuritis has also been associated with malignant diseases.[515] Johnson and colleagues[516] demonstrated that a clinical pattern of mononeuritis multiplex was the result of vasculitis of the nutrient vessels to the nerves. Two of their patients had unrecognized oat cell carcinomas of the lung. A third patient had a lymphoma and subsequently developed a liposarcoma. Again, the neurologic symptoms preceded the diagnosis of cancer by weeks to months.

PATHOPHYSIOLOGIC MECHANISMS

The existence of distinct tumor-associated antigens is well established.[517, 518] In this regard, circulating immune complexes can be detected in approximately one third to one half of cancer patients.[519, 520] The immune complexes are present in patients with both lymphoreticular and solid tumors. Tumor immune complex–mediated disease has been demonstrated in patients with Hodgkin's disease[518] and colon carcinoma.[517] Moreover, cryoglobulins can be demonstrated in some patients with lymphoma or multiple myeloma.[292] Circulating immune complexes were demonstrated in one patient with hairy cell leukemia and PAN[99] and were present in one patient with allergic angiitis associated with malignant melanoma (Cupps TR, and Fauci AS, unpublished observations). These observations at least suggest that immune complexes may play a significant role in the pathophysiology of the vasculitic syndromes seen in patients with cancer.

Studies conducted by Hellström et al.[521] and Ambrose et al.[522] have shown that circulating antibody is present when the tumor burden is small, such as in the early stages of tumor growth, during clinical remission, or following surgical removal. As the tumor burden increases, tumor-associated antigens increase and eventually produce a condition of antigen excess in which antibody directed against tumor antigen can no longer be detected.[522] Theoretically, at some point the condition of slight antigen excess is present, which may predispose to the formation of soluble circulating immune complexes with the potential for tissue deposition. This mechanism provides one plausible explanation for the observation that vasculitic symptoms frequently precede the diagnosis of tumor or closely follow treatment of cancer.

Additional mechanisms may be important in patients with hairy cell leukemia and PAN in which the vasculitis generally presents after the diagnosis of leukemia is made. Under these circumstances the reticuloendothelial system may be blocked by the neoplasm itself or by the tumor-released immune complexes. As a result, the blocked reticuloendothelial system may no longer be able to clear circulating complexes, which may then deposit in blood vessels and cause vasculitis. In this regard, clearance of heat-damaged erythrocytes was delayed in a single patient evaluated as having hairy cell leukemia and PAN.[128]

VASCULOPATHY ASSOCIATED WITH ATRIAL MYXOMA

The association between atrial myxoma and systemic vasculopathy has been emphasized.[199, 523-528] Strictly speaking, this syndrome is not a true vasculitis since the arterial lesions result from embolization of myxomatous tissue and subsequent invasion of the arterial wall.[523, 524, 527] However, discussion of this syndrome is appropriate because its clinical and angiographic presentation closely mimics that of true vasculitic syndromes.

Clinically, this disease may present with a picture of systemic vasculitis indistinguishable from PAN.[199, 527] CNS involvement is quite frequent, and a clinical picture of cerebral dysfunction similar to that seen in CNS vasculitis (see Chapter 10) may be the primary presenting symptom.[523-526]

Routine laboratory studies are nondiagnostic. Multiple arterial aneurysms can be seen on CNS or visceral angiographic studies.[199, 524, 526] The angiographic pattern seen is indistinguishable from that seen in classic PAN. With CNS involvement, cerebrospinal fluid analysis may be entirely normal or may demonstrate a mildly elevated protein.

The diagnosis is established by the finding of embolized myxomatous tissue on biopsy of an involved artery or by demonstration of an atrial filling defect on echocardiogram of the heart.

Treatment for this disease is surgical removal of the tumor. Unfortunately, the embolized material manifests local invasive properties.[523, 525] In this regard, a patient developed CNS involvement 3 years after surgical removal of an atrial myxoma.[528] Because of this observation, the prognosis of a patient with this syndrome is guarded. Early identification and removal of the tumor are suggested, and the need for additional therapy to treat the embolized tumor fragment should be evaluated. Currently, no data concerning treatment for the embolized tumor fragment are available.

SUMMARY

Systemic and cutaneous vasculitic syndromes, although rare, can be associated with neoplastic diseases. Frequently, the vasculitic syndrome precedes the diagnosis of tumor and may be the first sign of an occult neoplasm or the first evidence of recurrent disease. This pattern of the signs and symptoms of vasculitis preceding the signs and symptoms of the neoplasm appears to be particularly prevalent in patients with (1) Hodgkin's disease and CNS vasculitis, (2) solid tumors and extremity vasculitis, and (3) lymphoreticular neoplasms associated with hypersensitivity vasculitis.

In comparison, in the syndrome of hairy cell leukemia and PAN, the vasculitic component generally follows the diagnosis of the leukemia. Therefore, the clinician should closely evaluate symptoms that are not generally part of the hairy cell leukemia symptom complex. A high index of suspicion will help to establish the diagnosis of necrotizing vasculitis, perhaps thereby preventing morbid complications. Although treatment of the underlying neoplasm, if successful, may help resolve the vasculitic process, specific therapy for the necrotizing vasculitis may be necessary.

CHAPTER 10

CENTRAL NERVOUS SYSTEM VASCULITIS

INTRODUCTION

A wide variety of disease processes can produce vasculitis of the central nervous system (CNS). Because of the complexity and diversity of this topic, this chapter is divided into several sections. The first section focuses on isolated angiitis of the CNS. Subsequent sections discuss CNS vasculitis in relation to (1) infectious diseases, (2) rheumatic diseases, (3) systemic vasculitides, (4) neoplastic diseases, and (5) toxic agents. A final section briefly reviews a heterogeneous group of vasculopathies of the CNS that may or may not be related to a true vasculitic process.

ISOLATED ANGIITIS OF THE CNS (GRANULOMATOUS ANGIITIS OF THE CNS)

Definition. Isolated angiitis of the CNS is a distinct clinicopathologic entity characterized by vasculitis restricted to the vessels of the CNS.[509, 529-539] Most frequently it is associated with a granulomatous inflammatory process. Although the vessel most commonly affected is the arteriole, vessels of any size can be involved. The inflammatory infiltrate is usually composed of mononuclear cells with varying numbers of giant cells.

Pathophysiology. The etiology of isolated CNS angiitis is unknown. An association between a recent varicella-zoster infection and the development of granulomatous CNS angiitis has been observed.[505, 506, 540-544] Virus-like particles have been reported in samples of involved CNS tissue examined by electron microscopy by

123

some,[541, 544] but not all, authors.[506, 543] Other infectious agents, such as mycoplasma-like organisms, have also been suggested.[545] In this regard, isolated CNS vasculitis can be produced in turkeys by intravenous injection of *Mycoplasma gallisepticum*.[546] The disease process in turkeys appears to be a direct toxic effect rather than an immune-mediated problem.

The role of immune complexes in the pathogenesis of this disease has not been evaluated. The observation that nearly a quarter of patients with polyarteritis have CNS involvement suggests that immune complexes can produce disease in intracerebral vessels. In this regard, IgG deposition in the choroid plexus has been demonstrated in a patient with a systemic vasculitic process related to a prosthetic valve endocarditis.[534] Studies to investigate immune complex deposition in patients with isolated cerebral vasculitis have not been reported.

The unusual localization of the inflammatory process to intracerebral blood vessels is of interest. Factors at the level of the blood vessel may be important in this localization; for instance, anatomic changes such as the arteries entering the skull are well described.[535] In addition, functional characteristics such as the concept of the blood-brain barrier further differentiate the intracranial from the extracranial vessels. However, the true importance of these observations in relationship to the pathogenesis of isolated granulomatous angiitis of the CNS is unclear at present.

Incidence and prevalence. Isolated granulomatous angiitis of the CNS is a rare disease. If the cases associated with lymphoreticular tumors and systemic vasculitis are excluded, approximately 20 well-documented cases of this disease have been reported.[443, 509, 529-532, 536-539, 547-550] The majority of cases occur in the fifth to eighth decades, although the range extends from 2 to 96 years of age. The disease is seen in males and females with equal frequency.

Clinical manifestations. The most frequent initial symptoms are intellectual deterioration, confusion, headache, impaired consciousness, and nausea. Less frequently, seizure activity or spinal cord involvement is the initial symptom of disease. Progression to focal signs and symptoms such as hemiparesis or dysplasia is common. Evidence of cranial nerve involvement is seen at some point in the course of the disease in the majority of patients. Systemic symptoms such as fever, arthralgia, arthritis, and myalgia are uncommon.

Involvement of vessels in the spinal cord is seen in certain patients with intracranial disease.[530, 532] Several cases of isolated spinal cord vasculitis have been reported,[549, 550] including one associated with heroin drug abuse.[550]

Laboratory considerations. Routine laboratory studies are not particularly helpful. Frequently, early in the course of the disease, the erythrocyte sedimentation rate is normal. Cerebrospinal fluid (CSF) abnormalities include elevated opening pressure, mild pleocytosis (generally with a mononuclear pattern), and a mildly elevated protein. Higher levels of CSF protein are usually seen in patients with spinal cord involvement. Of note is the fact that, on the one hand, completely normal CSF studies have been reported[529, 547] and, on the other hand, findings suggesting intracranial hemorrhage can be seen.

Noninvasive studies of the CNS are for the most part nondiagnostic. Brain scans may be normal or may demonstrate areas of increased isotope uptake, depending on the disease activity at the time of the study. Similarly, studies with computed axial tomography can either be normal or demonstrate areas of decreased density. The electroencephalogram may show a seizure focus or a diffuse pattern of slowing.

In certain patients, cerebral angiography has proved most helpful in suggesting the diagnosis of angiitis. The most commonly described pattern is intermittent narrowing and dilatation of small vessels, resulting in a picture of "beading" of the vessels (Fig. 10–1). Involvement may be seen in the vessels around the base of the brain or in the more distal vessels.[533, 547] Other patterns, including displacement of small vessels, cut-off of vessels, and aneurysm formation, are less frequently noted. It should be emphasized that cerebral angiography may be entirely normal,[531, 539] reflecting involvement of much smaller vessels. Consequently, a negative study does *not* exclude the diagnosis.

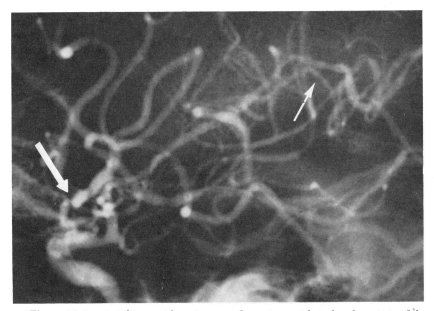

Figure 10–1. A right carotid angiogram of a patient with isolated angiitis of the central nervous system. Note the high-grade lesion in the proximal portion of the middle cerebral artery (large arrow) and a pattern of beading in the more distal vessels (small arrow).

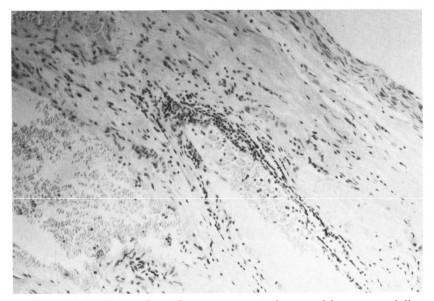

Figure 10–2. Biopsy of an inflammatory mass in the area of the conus medullaris and filum terminale of spinal canal in a patient with vasculitis isolated to the spinal cord. A mononuclear infiltration is present. Hematoxylin and eosin stain (original magnification ×130).

Pathology.   The pathologic pattern varies somewhat from case to case.[509, 529-539] Any CNS vessel may be involved, from the large intracranial arteries and veins to the capillaries and venules. The most frequently involved vessels, however, are the small arteries and precapillary arterioles. Although vessels in any area can be affected, angiitis of the leptomeningeal vessels is the most common finding.

The lesions are generally segmental and do not appear to have a predilection for bifurcation, as with the visceral vessel involvement of classic polyarteritis nodosa (PAN). The entire thickness of the vessels can be involved, although the greatest inflammatory response tends to be in the media or adventitia. The inflammatory infiltrate consists of mononuclear cells, including varying numbers of lymphocytes, monocytes, and histiocytes as well as plasma cells and giant cells (Fig. 10–2). Less frequently, areas of disruption of elastic membrane or necrosis of a vessel wall will be discerned. Areas with only perivascular cuffing or endothelial proliferation can also be identified.

Diagnosis and differential diagnosis.   The diagnosis of isolated angiitis of the CNS is difficult to establish. No single sign, symptom, or laboratory test establishes or rules out the diagnosis. Moreover, the diagnosis is one of exclusion, as a CNS vasculitic picture can be produced by a wide variety of diseases including syphilis, mycotic infections, tuberculosis, bacterial meningitis, rheumatic disease, systemic vasculitides, Hodgkin's disease, and atrial myxoma. The CSF findings are usually compatible with the diagnosis but are not themselves diagnostic. A pattern of beading or aneurysm in a cerebral angiogram can only suggest the diagnosis, since other causes of CNS vasculitis can produce a similar roentgenographic pattern. Also, a negative angiogram does not exclude the diagnosis, since in some patients only very small vessels are involved. Brain biopsies have been performed in an attempt to establish the diagnosis, but in one review[509] three of four tissue samples were nondiagnostic. Because of the frequent involvement of the leptomeningeal vessels, biopsy of this structure may prove to be more productive. Any tissue sample should be evaluated by special stains and culture to exclude infectious agents.

Isolated angiitis of the CNS should be included in the differential diagnosis of a CNS process when any of the following findings are present: (1) severe headache, (2) declining intellectual capacities, (3) altered mental status, (4) neurogenic emesis, (5) evidence for intracranial hemorrhage, (6) focal lesions, (7) cranial neuropathy, or (8) spinal cord obstruction. In any patient who presents with headache or impaired mental function or both and progresses to multifocal neurologic deficits without an established diagnosis, the possibility of isolated angiitis of the CNS should be aggressively evaluated.

Treatment and prognosis. Untreated, angiitis of the CNS is considered a fatal disease.[533] The clinical course varies with each case. A rapidly progressive course with a duration of days to weeks is seen in half the patients; in the remainder, a slower course with progression over months to years has been observed.[532]

The use of corticosteroids appears to improve clinical symptoms in some cases,[532] but progression of the disease during steroid therapy is well documented.[538, 547] A course of azathioprine did not appear to alter the course in one patient.[547] We have followed three patients with isolated granulomatous angiitis of the CNS (two with intracranial disease and one with spinal cord involvement) who have been stabilized on an immunosuppressive regimen of cyclophosphamide and alternate-day prednisone therapy for over 1 year. Further followup will be required to determine whether this regimen will produce sustained clinical remission.

DISEASES WITH WHICH CNS VASCULITIS CAN BE ASSOCIATED

INFECTIOUS DISEASES

Bacterial infections. Bacterial organisms may cause disease of CNS vessels by any of several mechanisms. An acute inflammatory process of the CNS vessels may be present in association with bacterial meningitis,[551, 552] with an acute inflammatory infiltrate extending to the subendothelial level.[552] This vascular involvement may be reflected in angiographic studies demonstrating symmetric narrowing of the large intracranial vessels at the base of the brain as well as narrowing or occlusion of smaller arteries.[551, 553, 554] The diagnosis can generally be established by appropriate studies, including culture of the CSF. Less frequently, localized infections of the cavernous sinus may produce mycotic aneurysms in adjacent intracranial vessels.[555] Septic emboli from endothelial infections such as endocarditis can produce mycotic aneurysms of CNS vessels. Rarely, symptoms from mycotic aneurysms may bring a patient to medical attention.[202] Generally, the diagnosis is established by cerebral angiography and appropriate CSF and blood cultures.

Abnormalities of the CNS vessels may be seen as a remote effect of bacterial infection without direct infection of intracranial structures. Abnormalities of CNS vessels have been described in patients with rheumatic fever who develop the associated chorea.[556] The pathogenesis of this abnormality is not fully understood.

Syphilis. Tertiary syphilis can produce a CNS arteritis. Although in the majority of cases the primary site is the leptomeningeal vessels, involvement of other intracranial vessels can be seen. Involvement of the larger vessels can be demonstrated with angiographic studies showing narrowing of the vessels.[557, 558] The clinical presentation can be varied but includes altered higher cortical function as well as evidence of focal abnormalities. The diagnosis is established with the appropriate serologic studies of blood and CSF.

Tuberculosis. Tuberculous meningitis can produce a vasculitis of large intracranial arteries.[559, 560] Histologically, the pattern of acute and chronic inflammation with endothelial proliferation can be seen, with particularly severe involvement of the vessels at the base of the brain. The pathologic process is reflected in angiographic studies, which demonstrate irregularity and narrowing of the carotid artery as it enters the cranial vault. Narrowing of more distal arteries, such as the anterior cerebral or middle cerebral arteries, may also be present.[560] Clinically, symptoms of cerebral dysfunction resulting from the compromised perfusion of the middle cerebral artery are most commonly seen.

In addition, a small vessel vasculitis with vessel infiltration by mononuclear cells can also occur in association with tuberculosis.[561] The size of the vessel involved is beyond the resolution of angiographic studies, although evidence of a mass lesion may be present.

Fungal infections. Two types of mycotic arteritis have been described, the tuberculous and the hyphal types.[562] The tuberculous type presents as a basilar meningitis, producing vasculitis of large intracranial arteries at the base of the brain. The infections that produce this type of mycotic arteritis include coccidioidomycosis, actinomycosis, cryptococcosis, histoplasmosis, and nocardiosis. The hyphal type presents with tangles of hyphae in the vessel lumina and is produced by the organisms that cause aspergillosis, candidiasis, and phycomycosis, including mucormycosis.

Direct invasion of the vessels by *Aspergillus* organisms has produced thromboendoarteritis of the carotid, anterior cerebral, and middle cerebral arteries.[563, 564] Mycotic aneurysm formation leading to subarachnoid hemorrhage has also been reported in *Aspergillus* infections.[565]

Cerebral mucormycosis, because of its vascular invasive tendencies, can also produce devastating disease.[566-568] The clinical presentation of eye involvement in the setting of acidosis, as seen in poorly controlled diabetes mellitus, has been emphasized. The angiographic picture reflects the invasion of vessels with a pattern of stenosis, occlusion, and embolism.[569]

Viral infections. The association between CNS angiitis and varicella-zoster virus has been mentioned previously. Patients with Hodgkin's disease who develop CNS angiitis frequently have an associated herpes zoster infection.[505, 506, 544] Cases of CNS angiitis associated with varicella-zoster infection in the absence of lymphoreticular neoplasm have also been reported.[540-543]

Angiographic studies in these patients generally show a pattern of beading and narrowing of the intracerebral arteries. The histologic pattern is a panarteritis with a predominantly mononuclear cell infiltrate.[541] Giant cells are seen with varying frequency.

Virus-like particles have been reported in electron microscopic studies around the vessels by some,[541, 544] but not all, observers.[506, 543] Attempts to culture the virus from brain tissue have not been successful. Finally, it should be noted that neurologic dysfunction associated with varicella-zoster infections of the trigeminal nerve may result from mechanisms other than CNS vasculitis.[570]

Other infectious organisms. Thomas et al.[546] produced cerebral vasculitis in turkeys using intravenous injections of *Mycoplasma gallisepticum*. The syndrome was prevented by treatment with antibiotics, such as tetracycline, but was not altered by immunosuppressive agents, such as corticosteroids or methotrexate. This observation suggests a direct toxic effect rather than an immune-mediated mechanism for this particular type of animal model vasculitis. Mycoplasma-like structures have been reported in electron microscopic studies done on tissue from a patient with CNS angiitis.[545] The significance of this observation is unclear and remains to be determined. Finally, a clinical picture of self-limited CNS angiitis has been reported in association with cat-scratch disease.[571]

Rheumatic Disorders

Systemic lupus erythematosus (SLE). CNS involvement plays a major role in the clinical spectrum of SLE.[572, 573] Cerebral dysfunction in SLE can be caused by large vessel or by small vessel involvement or by both. In addition, a condition of "cerebritis" may be present, which is apparently unrelated to vascular involvement. No satisfactory anatomic lesion has been defined for "cerebritis," and the pathophysiology is poorly understood.

Large vessel intracranial arteritis in SLE is a well-established syndrome.[574] Clinically, the syndrome presents most frequently with a hemiparesis reflecting the frequent involvement of the internal carotid and middle cerebral arteries.[574] CSF findings are nondiagnostic and may even be normal.[574] The angiographic studies demonstrate narrowing or occlusion of large intracranial arteries.[574] The vasculitic nature of this process has been demonstrated histopathologically as an acute inflammatory infiltrate and necrosis.[572]

Other, more focal lesions can be caused by lupus CNS vasculitis and include the development of chorea[575] and visual abnormalities.[576] Vasculitic lesions may be responsible for at least some cases of transverse myelopathy seen in SLE.[577] Moreover, in patients with SLE who exhibited psychiatric symptoms, evidence of systemic vasculitis was much more frequent.[573] This observation suggests that some of the varied symptoms of higher cortical dysfunction could be related to small vessel CNS disease. The relative importance of small vessel vasculitis and "cerebritis" in the CNS disease of SLE cannot be accurately evaluated because currently, short of an autopsy examination, the two syndromes cannot be clinically distinguished.

Other rheumatic disorders. Any of the collagen, vascular, or rheumatic diseases that have been associated with PAN (see Table 4–7) may include a picture of CNS vasculitis. Isolated CNS vasculitis with rheumatoid arthritis is a well-established association.[578-581] In isolated CNS vasculitis with rheumatoid arthritis, the presenting symptoms may be related to an intracranial hemorrhage.[580] The disorder is a necrotizing vasculitis of small- and intermediate-sized intracranial arteries.[579] An association with amyloid deposits has been noted.[578, 581] Isolated cerebral artery involvement has also been reported in patients with scleroderma.[582, 583]

Systemic Vasculitides

As noted in preceding chapters, the major systemic vasculitic syndromes can also involve CNS vessels. In autopsy studies, over a quarter of patients with systemic necrotizing vasculitis have involvement of CNS vessels (see Table 2–5). In this group, CNS vasculitis was the apparent cause of death in 15 per cent of patients (see Table 2–4). Angiographic findings include vessel narrowing, dilatations, and aneurysm formation.[108, 584]

In Wegener's granulomatosis, CNS vasculitis does not appear to be as frequent as in the other systemic vasculitides, but well-documented cases of necrotizing vasculitis of the intracranial arteries have been reported.[358] In comparison, CNS involvement is more frequent in lymphomatoid granulomatosis, in which vasculitis of the intracranial vessels is well established.[585] Rarely, vasculitis of small CNS vessels is present in systemic hypersensitivity angiitis syndromes, such as Henoch-Schönlein purpura.[247]

NEOPLASMS

Hodgkin's disease associated with CNS granulomatous angiitis and the vasculopathy associated with atrial myxoma have been discussed in Chapter 9. It is important to note that both syndromes may present primarily with CNS-related symptoms, thus concealing the associated neoplastic disease. Direct invasion of vessels by a variety of CNS tumors can produce an irregular or "shaggy" pattern on angiographic studies,[586, 587] mimicking a pattern seen in vasculitis.

TOXIC OR METABOLIC ABNORMALITIES

The association of necrotizing vasculitis, particularly of the CNS, with the abuse of amphetamines has been reported.[185, 588] The histologic picture is similar to that of the necrotizing vasculitis seen in PAN. Angiographic changes include the pattern of focal narrowing and widening of vessels with a "beaded" appearance. Intracerebral hemorrhage has also been reported.[588]

Vascular occlusion has rarely been reported following CNS radiation for tumor.[589, 590] The histologic lesion is characterized by marked endothelial proliferation associated with foam cells. Cerebral vasculitis has been described with the use of allopurinol in a patient with partial hypoxanthine-guanine phosphoribosyl transferase deficiency.[591] The mechanism for this reaction is unclear.

MISCELLANEOUS VASCULOPATHIES

There are several other disease processes that involve vessels in the CNS. The pathophysiology of these entities is not understood and is not necessarily associated with vascular inflammation.

A poorly defined syndrome of internal carotid or middle cerebral artery occlusion in children or young adults has been described.[592-595] The clinical presentation results from hypoperfusion in the distribution of the middle cerebral artery. Although the majority of cases were associated with trauma[593, 594] in the region of the carotid artery, some of the cases were preceded by a severe infection, including upper respiratory tract infection, otitis, pharyngitis, and tonsillitis.[593] In these latter cases, direct extension of the inflammatory process from the infected focus may have produced a carotid arteritis with subsequent vascular occlusion.[592]

A syndrome of spontaneous, gradual occlusion of the circle of Willis is a rare disease seen in people of Japanese ancestry.[596, 597] The term "moyamoya" has been applied to the syndrome. This Japanese word describes "something hazy like a puff of cigarette smoke drifting in the air" and is applied to the net-like pattern of collateral vessels seen on cerebral angiography.[597] A pediatric form of "moyamoya" is characterized by recurrent episodes of hemiplegia, while the adult form is associated with altered mental status and subarachnoid hemorrhage.[597] The ESR and CSF evaluations are generally normal. The diagnosis is established by the characteristic pattern seen on cerebral angiography. The etiology of the disease is unclear, and no effective therapy has been established.

Rarely, other diseases may be associated with occlusions of intracranial vessels. This finding may be present in patients with thrombotic thrombocytopenic purpura.[598, 599] Occlusion of large cerebral vessels may be seen in patients with sickle cell anemia.[600] The etiology of the abnormality is unknown, but vascular ischemia secondary to sickling in the vasa vasorum has been suggested. Occlusions of large vessels in the CNS have also been described in neurofibromatosis.[601]

CHAPTER 11

THROMBOANGIITIS OBLITERANS (BUERGER'S DISEASE, ENDARTERITIS OBLITERANS)

Definition. Thromboangiitis obliterans is an inflammatory occlusive vascular disease involving intermediate- to small-sized arteries and veins of the extremities.[602-606] The disease is seen predominantly in males who have a significant smoking history.

Pathophysiology. The etiology of thromboangiitis obliterans is unknown. Reports evaluating immunologic function in patients with this disease have not demonstrated a uniform pattern of abnormalities. In one study,[607] immunoglobulin levels, complement levels, and numbers of B and T lymphocytes were all normal, although 35 per cent of patients had detectable antibodies against heat-denatured human collagen. In comparison,[608] another study of patients with thromboangiitis obliterans demonstrated elevated immunoglobulins and cryoglobulins, depressed complement levels, and inhibited leukocyte migration after exposure to arterial antigen. Clearly, further definition of immune-related events in this disease is needed.

The frequent association of thrombosis and thrombophlebitis with thromboangiitis obliterans has lead to an evaluation of the clotting system in patients with this disease. Increased platelet adhesion was reported in patients with thromboangiitis obliterans, but the values decreased significantly toward normal when the patients stopped smoking.[609] The significance of this observation is unclear, because the adhesive platelet count was also elevated in patients with thrombophlebitis not associated with thromboangiitis

133

obliterans. An increased level of heparin-precipitable fraction of fibrinogen has also been reported in a group of patients with thromboangiitis obliterans.[610]

Genetic factors appear to be important in the pathogenesis of thromboangiitis obliterans. An increased incidence of the disease is seen in Oriental populations[604, 605] and Ashkenazi Jews in Israel.[606] Also, HLA antigens A9 and B5 are more frequent, and B12 less frequent, in patients with thromboangiitis obliterans when compared with a normal control population.[611, 612]

The role of environmental factors, particularly cigarette smoking, is emphasized in virtually all major reports on this disease. Cessation of smoking generally results in stabilization of the disease process. Other factors including trauma, exposure to cold, particularly the development of frostbite, and fungal infections of the feet have been recorded in association with thromboangiitis obliterans.[604, 605, 613] The importance of these observations to the pathogenesis of this disease is unclear.

Incidence and prevalence. Thromboangiitis obliterans is a rare disease, but no true incidence or prevalence has been determined. Two striking features are the male predominance, which exceeds the ratio of 9 to 1, and the onset of symptoms before the age of 40 years in the vast majority of patients.

Clinical considerations. The most common presenting symptom, seen in approximately 40 per cent of cases, is claudication of a lower extremity.[606] Migratory thrombophlebitis is the initial symptom in over a quarter of patients. Less frequently, presenting signs and symptoms include numbness, pain, ulceration, or infection of the toes. Of note, less than 5 per cent of patients present with symptoms related to the upper extremities.[606]

Clinical symptoms that persist throughout the course of the disease are strikingly similar to the presenting symptoms. Migratory thrombophlebitis, usually in multiple episodes, is seen in 60 per cent of patients. Raynaud's phenomenon is present in greater than 50 per cent of patients, and hyperhydrosis occurs in a third of patients. In contrast to the findings described at presentation, greater than 90 per cent of patients will have involvement of the upper extremities at some stage of the disease. Although the disease is generally restricted to the extremities, vessels in the head, heart, viscera, and epididymis may occasionally be involved.[605, 606, 614, 615] Systemic symptoms such as fever, malaise, myalgias, or arthralgias are generally absent.

Laboratory considerations. Routine laboratory studies are not particularly helpful in establishing the diagnosis. The erythrocyte sedimentation rate (ESR) may be normal, and serum lipids are not generally elevated. Serologic studies such as antinuclear antibody or rheumatoid factor tend to be negative.

In contrast, angiography of involved extremities can provide important diagnostic clues.[605, 606] The earliest angiographic evidence of thromboangiitis obliterans is most often found in the arteries of the feet. When there is involvement of the upper extremity, occlusion of the ulnar or radial artery at the wrist is common. Tortuosity of an artery, such as the radial artery, reflects the recanalization of the vessel. The digital arteries may be pruned or cut while the interosseous arteries are spared.[605] Similar findings can be appreciated in studies of the lower extremities. The segmental nature of the disease is characterized by a pattern of abrupt symmetric tapering. In addition, multiple small arteries may be demonstrated in an area of obstruction producing a "spider legs" or "root" pattern.[605] In contrast to the segmental symmetric narrowing seen in thromboangiitis obliterans, atherosclerotic vessels tend to have an asymmetric, diffuse pattern.

Pathology. The vascular lesions of thromboangiitis obliterans tend to involve intermediate and small arteries and veins of the extremities. The lesions are segmental in nature and may be in any stage of evolution at any given time. The histopathology has been divided into three stages — acute, subacute, and chronic.[604-606, 616] The *acute stage* is characterized by an inflammatory infiltration of the vessel wall with polymorphonuclear cells. Invariably there is a thrombus associated with the vascular lesion, and pockets of polymorphonuclear cells forming microabscesses may be present within the thrombus. It should be emphasized that vessel integrity, including the elastic membrane, remains intact. In the *subacute stage,* mononuclear cells predominate and giant cells may be present in varying numbers. The *chronic stage* is characterized by fibrosis and recanalization of the thrombus.

Diagnosis and differential diagnosis. Thromboangiitis obliterans needs to be distinguished from atherosclerosis obliterans. Thromboangiitis as a clinical entity separate from atherosclerosis had been challenged in the past,[617, 618] but subsequent studies[604-606] reported pathologic, angiographic, and epidemiologic criteria that clearly establish thromboangiitis obliterans as a distinct entity. The diagnosis is established by biopsy of an involved artery or by angiography. In addition, diseases associated with Raynaud's phenomenon, such as systemic lupus erythematosus, scleroderma, and other systemic vasculitides, should be excluded. Finally, the diagnosis of thromboangiitis obliterans should be included in the differential diagnosis of migratory thrombophlebitis, particularly if the upper extremities are involved.

Treatment and prognosis. Although morbidity in the form of tissue or extremity loss may be extensive, long-term survival is not significantly altered. Cessation of smoking and meticulous care of an ischemic extremity during an acute exacerbation are basic in the treatment of this disease. The role of reconstructive vascular surgery is limited.[619-621] Bypass grafting of a single large obstructed artery appears to have the best chance for a good clinical outcome. Attempts at thromboendarterectomy have been uniformly unsuccessful. Other therapies, including induced hypertension[622] and intravenous prostaglandin E_1,[623] have also been tried with limited success.

CHAPTER 12

MUCOCUTANEOUS LYMPH NODE SYNDROME (KAWASAKI DISEASE)

Definition. Mucocutaneous lymph node syndrome (MLNS), or Kawasaki disease, is an acute illness of infants and young children characterized by (1) sustained fever, (2) bilateral congestion of the ocular conjunctivae, (3) changes in the lips and oral mucosa, (4) changes in the peripheral extremities, (5) nonvesicular truncal exanthem, and (6) acute nonsuppurative enlargement of the cervical lymph nodes.[624, 625] The disease course is usually self-limited, although a small number (1 to 2 per cent) of cases are fatal owing to sudden death from coronary arteritis, which is similar, if not identical, in pattern to infantile polyarteritis nodosa (PAN).[626]

Pathophysiology. The etiology of MLNS is unknown. Several different infectious agents have been suggested as potential pathogens, although none has been consistently implicated. Rickettsia-like bodies have been demonstrated on electron microscopic studies of involved lymph nodes.[627] Epstein-Barr virus[628] and streptococcal bacteria[629] have also been implicated in isolated cases. A role for immune complexes has been suggested,[630, 631] although studies demonstrating immune complex deposition in involved tissues are lacking.

A genetic or environmental factor is suggested by the relatively high frequency of this disease in Japan, with thousands of cases having been reported.[626] In Hawaii, the incidence of MLNS was significantly greater in patients of Japanese ancestry than in those with a Caucasian background.[632] No high- or low-frequency HLA marker has been recognized in association with MLNS.[633]

137

TABLE 12-1. CLINICAL MANIFESTATIONS OF MLNS°

MANIFESTATIONS	PERCENTAGE
Fever	95
Changes of the extremity	
Desquamation from finger tips	94
Erythematous palms and soles	88
Indurated edema	76
Polymorphous exanthem of body and trunk	92
Changes in lips and oral cavity	
Dry, red lips	90
Erythematous oral mucosa	90
Prominent tongue papillae	77
Congested conjunctivae	88
Swelling of cervical nodes	75

°Data are summarized from 760 patients reported in reference 624.

Incidence and prevalence. Epidemiologic data on MLNS from Japan and the United States are variable.[625] Thousands of cases have been seen in Japan, and increasing numbers of cases are being reported in the United States.[634] The male to female ratio in the United States is 1.5 to 1, which is similar to the Japanese experience. The mean age at onset for confirmed cases in the United States is 3.8 years with a range of from 3 months to 13 years, which is higher than the mean age of approximately 1 year in Japan.

Clinical considerations. The clinical manifestations of MLNS have been previously reviewed in detail[624-626] and are summarized in Table 12-1.

FEVER. An elevated temperature is present in the vast majority of patients and varies in the range of 38 to 39° C. The temperature generally remains elevated for several days to weeks and is unresponsive to antibiotic therapy. Resolution of the fever generally occurs during the second week of illness.

EXTREMITIES. The initial sign in the extremities is a pronounced reddening of the palms and soles during the first week of the illness. Toward the end of the first week a nonpitting indurated edema of the distal extremities may also be present. During the second week of illness as the fever abates, a membranous desquamation begins at the finger tips.

EXANTHEM. The maculopapular eruption starts at approximately the third to fifth day and may progress to confluent lesions with resolution by the end of the first week of illness. Vesiculation or crusting is not seen.

HEAD AND NECK. Dry erythematous lips and oral mucosa and congested conjunctivae are characteristic during the first week of the disease. Prominent tongue papillae may produce a strawberry-like appearance. Nonsuppurative cervical lymphadenopathy is present in 75 per cent of cases.

LESS COMMON MANIFESTATIONS. Less frequently, signs and symptoms of cardiac dysfunction may start during the acute phase of the illness and reflect complications of the pancarditis that may be part of MLNS. Signs and symptoms of congestive heart failure may result from a myocardiopathy or valvular lesions such as mitral[635-637] or, less frequently, aortic[638] insufficiency. Delayed cardiac events are generally related to complications from coronary arteritis, often with resulting coronary artery aneurysms.[626, 639-641] Although coronary aneurysms can be demonstrated in nearly 20 per cent of patients with MLNS,[640] the mortality is less than 2 per cent.[626] The most common fatal lesion is a thrombus in an aneurysm with occlusion of the coronary artery and tissue infarction. Less frequently, a ruptured coronary aneurysm may produce fatal pericardial tamponade, or rupture of an aneurysm at another site may cause a fatal hemorrhage. Other unusual manifestations include diarrhea, arthralgia, arthritis, urethritis, aseptic meningitis, focal encephalopathy, and mild jaundice.[642]

Laboratory considerations. Leukocytosis with a shift toward less mature granulocyte forms is frequently present. During the acute phase of the disease, the erythrocyte sedimentation rate is elevated. Elevation of serum IgE levels, with a peak between the first and second week, has been reported.[96] The elevated IgE level returns to normal in 1 to 2 months.

Because mortality is most commonly related to cardiac events, evaluation of the heart has received emphasis. An electrocardiogram may be abnormal during the acute phase of the illness in the presence of myocarditis but tends to normalize as the disease resolves, even in the presence of coronary artery aneurysms. Coronary angiograms are useful to document the presence of aneurysms. However, owing to the low proportion of cardiac complications among the total group of patients with MLNS, this invasive procedure should not be used routinely. It should be reserved for patients in whom coronary artery disease is strongly suspected. Recently, the use of the noninvasive technique of two-dimensional echocardiography to diagnose coronary aneurysms has been emphasized.[643-645]

Pathology. The spectrum of histologic findings in MLNS has been reviewed in detail[626, 646-648] and in most cases reflects the findings at autopsy. The primary pathology is panangiitis of the coronary arteries. The inflammatory infiltrate is composed primarily of mononuclear cells, including lymphocytes and histiocytes. Disruption of the elastic membrane, areas of necrosis, and aneurysm formation are found in the areas of severe involvement. Endothelial proliferation is commonly seen, and giant cells are generally *not* present. Involvement of veins appears to be uncommon.

Again, the coronary arteries are the most common site of disease, with virtually 100 per cent involvement.[626, 648] Severe panangiitis can also be found in iliac arteries.[648] Involvement of other sites, including the aortic, celiac, carotid, subclavian, and pulmonary arteries, occurs less frequently, and histologic changes are generally restricted to endothelial proliferation.[648]

Histologic findings at sites other than arteries are less frequently described.[626, 646] The heart may show evidence of endocarditis, or myocarditis with myocardial histiocytes in areas of infarction. Findings in involved lymph nodes include local necrosis, small thrombi, inflammation of small vessels, and the presence of immunoblast-like cells.[626]

The similarity of the histologic findings in patients with a syndrome of infantile PAN (see Chapter 4) and in the fatal cases of MLNS has been emphasized.[626, 649-651] It is now generally felt that many of the cases of "infantile PAN" with coronary arteritis and a high fatality rate in fact represented the most severe expression of MLNS in infants.

Diagnosis and differential diagnosis. The diagnosis is based on the clinical presentation. If five of the six characteristic findings as listed in the definition are present, the diagnosis of MLNS is established.[626] The differential diagnosis of MLNS would include scarlet fever, meningococcemia, systemic lupus erythematosus, Stevens-Johnson syndrome, juvenile rheumatoid arthritis, scleroderma, viral syndromes, and Rocky Mountain spotted fever.[652] Recently, cases of MLNS in young adults have been reported,[653-656] but care should be taken to exclude the toxic shock syndrome.[657] The presence of hypotension, azotemia, and thrombocytopenia suggests the diagnosis of toxic shock syndrome as opposed to MLNS.

With regard to the initial manifestations of MLNS, if the diagnosis is considered, it is usually not difficult to make, given the characteristic features of the disease. However, great difficulty is often encountered in determining the approach and extent of diagnostic work-up that should be undertaken to establish the presence of cardiac complications, which may abruptly appear during the convalescent period and result in sudden death. Since the proportion of cardiac complications is so low, routine invasive procedures are out of the question. Although the optimal approach to this problem has not yet been established, investigators are currently employing noninvasive cardiac diagnostic techniques, such as two-dimensional echocardiography and isotope scanning techniques, in patients in whom there is a suspicion of impending cardiac complications.

Treatment and prognosis. Except for the 1 to 2 per cent of cases with a fatal outcome from cardiac complications, MLNS is a self-limited disease with a full functional recovery.[625, 626] Of the patients with a fatal outcome, the mortality rates are 50 per cent in 1 month, 75 per cent in 2 months, and 90 per cent in 6 months.[641] Rarely, complications of coronary artery involvement will follow the acute febrile episode by years.[658, 659]

Aspirin, 30 mg per kg per day in divided doses, appears to be the treatment of choice during the acute phase.[660] Antibiotic therapy does not appear to alter the course of the illness and corticosteroids may predispose to aneurysm formation.[660] In selected patients with cardiac lesions, coronary artery bypass grafting[658, 659] or valvuloplasty[636] may be indicated.

CHAPTER 13

BEHÇET'S DISEASE

Definition. Behçet's disease is a clinicopathologic entity characterized by recurrent episodes of oral ulcers, eye lesions, genital ulcers, and other cutaneous lesions.[661-664] The underlying pathologic lesion is a vasculitis involving predominantly venules, although vessels of any size in any organ system can be affected.[663, 664]

Pathophysiology. The etiology of Behçet's disease is unknown, but various possible causes, such as viral, immune-mediated, and genetic, have been suggested. Behçet's original proposal that the disease is caused by a virus[664] prompted numerous attempts to isolate an infectious agent; however, reports citing virus isolation[665-667] have been indecisive. Furthermore, a subsequent attempt to isolate a virus was unproductive.[668, 669]

Immune-mediated abnormalities have also been proposed. Circulating immune complexes demonstrated by the Raji cell assay and tissue deposition of immunoglobulin and complement components shown by immunofluorescence[670] suggest that immune complexes may play a role in the pathogenesis of Behçet's disease.[670] Lymphocyte-mediated cytotoxicity of oral epithelial cells has been noted in patients with active Behçet's disease.[671] The significance of this observation with respect to the pathophysiology of Behçet's disease is unclear, because cytotoxicity against oral epithelial cells is also seen in patients with recurrent aphthous stomatitis during periods of increased disease activity, and is hence not specific for Behçet's disease.

The increased incidence of Behçet's disease in eastern Mediterranean[663] and Far Eastern countries[664] suggests that environmental or genetic considerations may be important. An increased incidence of a genetic histocompatibility marker, HLA-B5, has been demonstrated in patients with Behçet's disease[672, 673]; furthermore, there appears to be an association of an HLA genetic marker with the clinical subtypes of the syndrome, such as the association of HLA-B5 with ocular, HLA-B27 with arthritic, and HLA-B12 with mucocutaneous disease patterns.[673]

Incidence and prevalence. Incidence and prevalence data are difficult to assess because of the apparent variations in date, location, and ethnic background. A range in prevalence from 1 per 10,000 to 1 per 300,000 has been reported (reviewed in reference 664). The marked male predominance (approximately 5 to 1) noted in series from the eastern Mediterranean countries[663, 674, 675] has not been found in smaller series in the United States,[676] where the ratio is closer to 1 to 1. The reasons for these observed variations are unclear.

Clinical manifestations. The following discussion on clinical manifestations largely reflects the experience of Chajek and Fainaru,[663] summarized in Table 13–1, and a review by Shimizu et al.[664] The earliest clinical manifestation of Behçet's disease, seen in nearly 75 per cent of patients, is oral ulceration. Ocular and joint symptoms are the earliest manifestations in approximately 10 per cent of patients. The symptoms that most commonly bring the patient to the attention of a physician, however, are the ocular and oral lesions, each of which is found in 25 per cent of presenting patients. Thrombophlebitis, joint symptoms, and neuropsychiatric problems each account for an additional 10 per cent. Less frequently, skin problems or genital ulcers are presenting symptoms.

*TABLE 13–1.   CLINICAL MANIFESTATIONS OF BEHÇET'S DISEASE**

MANIFESTATION	PERCENTAGE
Oral ulcers	98
Genital ulcers	88
Cutaneous lesions (excluding genital ulcers)	88
Pustules and pyoderma	46
Papules and vesicles	34
Erythema nodosum	32
Ocular dysfunction	76
Anterior chamber	66
Posterior structures	44
Thrombophlebitis	37
Superficial	27
Deep	24
Following venipuncture	12
Neurologic dysfunction	29
Joint symptoms	29

*Data are summarized from 41 patients reported in reference 663.

ORAL ULCERS. The oral lesion, which appears singly or in crops, starts as a slightly raised, reddened area and progresses to a shallow, "punched-out" ulcer 2 to 10 mm in diameter with a yellowish necrotic base. The ulcer, which may be quite painful, tends to resolve over 1 to 2 weeks. The most common sites of involvement are the lips, gingivae, buccal mucosa, and tongue. Structures in the posterior pharynx are less frequently affected.

GENITAL ULCERS. The genital lesions closely resemble the oral ulcers both in appearance and in clinical course. The most common site is on the scrotum in males and on the vulva in females. Less frequently, the skin of the penis and the vaginal mucosa may be involved. The lesions tend to be more symptomatic in males. Healing with scar tissue formation is more common with the genital lesions.

CUTANEOUS LESIONS. A wide variety of cutaneous lesions, including pustules, pyoderma, papules, vesicles, erythema nodosum, folliculitis, furuncles, and abscesses, have been associated with Behçet's disease. Increased skin reactivity to minor trauma such as a scratch or a superficial injection has also been noted.

OCULAR SYMPTOMS. The most common site of involvement is in the anterior chamber with a pattern of iridocyclitis and hypopyon. The lesion is usually transient, with resolution in several days and no apparent long-term sequelae. In the posterior ocular structures, chemical manifestations include choroiditis, retinal vessel arteritis or phlebitis, optic papillitis, and vitreous involvement. Recurrent attacks in the posterior structures characteristically lead to blindness in 5 to 6 years. Glaucoma and cataract formation may also complicate the clinical picture.

THROMBOPHLEBITIS. Recurrent thrombophlebitis of both the deep and the superficial venous systems is seen in approximately a third of patients. The episodes of thrombophlebitis are associated with the systemic signs of fever and prostration, which may persist despite standard anticoagulant therapy. The development of phlebitis following an uncomplicated venipuncture strongly suggests the possibility of Behçet's disease. Even intravenous heparin may cause a local superficial thrombophlebitis.[624] Obstruction of the inferior or superior vena cava is a not infrequent complication of this disease.

NEUROLOGIC DYSFUNCTION. Although present in only a minority of patients, neurologic involvement has received considerable attention because of its associated high mortality.[677, 678] Essentially any pattern of neurologic dysfunction may be present, but the most common presentations are hemiplegia, severe headaches, hyperesthesia, and paraplegia.[664] In addition, patterns of cranial nerve palsy, cerebellar dysfunction, meningoencephalitis, altered mood, and mental status changes have been noted. The neurologic complications of Behçet's disease generally occur late, with a mean of 7 years after the first evidence of disease.[663] Significant recovery is generally seen, but recurrent episodes may result in major neurologic deficits.

JOINTS. True arthritis is usually seen in association with other manifestations of Behçet's disease. The most commonly involved joint is the knee, although the elbow or the wrist may also be affected. Despite recurrent arthritic attacks, joint deformity is not seen.

KIDNEYS. Renal involvement, originally thought to be rare,[663] may in fact be common.[679, 680] Over a third of patients in one series[680] had proteinuria or hematuria or both. Renal lesions may be caused by a glomerulonephritis[670] or an infiltration by amyloid.[679] Progression to functional renal impairment is not characteristic of Behçet's syndrome. Rarely, a patient will develop urethritis or epididymitis.

CARDIOVASCULAR SYSTEM. Cardiac involvement is generally limited to pericarditis, which is seen in an occasional case.[681] Aneurysm formation or large artery occlusion can be seen in some cases and may result in a fatal outcome.[664]

PULMONARY SYSTEM. Problems related to the lungs appear to be relatively uncommon in Behçet's disease.[682] However, if pulmonary involvement does occur, it may be dramatic, such as life-threatening pulmonary hemorrhage. An association between superior vena cava obstruction and pulmonary hemorrhage has been noted.[682]

GASTROINTESTINAL TRACT. Symptoms related to the gastrointestinal tract are not unusual in Behçet's disease.[664] Ulcers have been demonstrated from the esophagus[683] to the rectum, although the most frequent sites of involvement are the ileum and cecum.[664] Perforation of the abdominal viscus may lead to life-threatening complications.

Laboratory considerations. Routine laboratory studies done during an active episode of disease generally demonstrate a leukocytosis and an elevated erythrocyte sedimentation rate. Immunoglobulin levels may be elevated, but serum complement levels are generally normal. Decreased plasma fibrinolytic activity has been reported.[663] Cerebrospinal fluid studies during an active episode involving the central nervous system (CNS) may show a moderately elevated protein and a mild to moderate pleocytosis composed either of mononuclear cells or of polymorphonuclear cells.

Pathology. The underlying pathologic lesion appears to be a vasculitis.[664, 684] Small vessel involvement predominates, with a mononuclear cell infiltrate. Frequently, there is a perivascular pattern and thrombosis. Endothelial proliferation or necrosis is less frequently seen. Even when large vessels are involved, the primary site of pathology may be the vasa vasorum.[664] Biopsies of oral lesions may or may not demonstrate a vasculitis, but a mononuclear cell infiltrate is characteristic.[684] However, giant cells are not characteristically seen.

Diagnosis. Behçet's disease is a clinicopathologic diagnosis. Not infrequently, definitive diagnosis eludes the clinician owing to the fact that there are no absolute diagnostic findings. Specifically, the diagnosis of Behçet's syndrome is established by major clinical criteria, which include: (1) recurrent oral ulcers; (2) skin lesions, including erythema nodosum–like lesions, subcutaneous thrombophlebitis, and hyperreactivity of the skin; (3) eye lesions, including iridocyclitis and chorioretinitis; and (4) genital ulcerations.[664] The diagnosis is established not upon presentation of the first symptoms, but when three of the four major criteria are present. Generally, the life-threatening complications, such as neurologic dysfunction or gastrointestinal tract involvement, occur late in the course of the disease after the diagnosis is apparent.

Treatment and prognosis. There is no uniformly satisfactory therapy for Behçet's disease.[663, 664, 685] Consequently, a large number of agents have been tried with varying degrees of success. An initial observation of clinical improvement following blood transfusion[676] was not subsequently confirmed.[686] Trials of transfer factor demonstrated improvement in some cases.[687] Chemotherapeutic agents, such as phenformin and ethylestrenol, which increase the blood fibrinolytic activity, have been used, particularly in the setting of ongoing complications related to thrombophlebitis.[688] Because of increased chemotactic activity of polymorphonuclear cells in Behçet's disease, colchicine has been tried,[689, 690] with a successful experience reported. A preliminary report suggests that levamisole may also be useful in this disease.[691] Corticosteroids, both topically and systemically, may suppress symptoms but do not appear to alter the course of the underlying disease. Nonsteroidal anti-inflammatory agents, such as indomethacin, have also been tried with limited success.[681] Immunosuppressive drugs, including cyclophosphamide, azathioprine, and chlorambucil, have been used with a reported favorable response.[692-695] However, there are no adequately controlled trials to demonstrate efficacy of one agent over another.

In the absence of CNS, bowel, or large artery involvement, the prognosis for life is good. The need for early, aggressive treatment of CNS disease has been stressed.[678] Involvement of the posterior structures of the eye has been relatively refractory to therapy; consequently, the long-term prognosis for useful vision is guarded in patients with serious ocular involvement.

CHAPTER 14

MISCELLANEOUS SYNDROMES

INTRODUCTION

Several miscellaneous vasculitic syndromes, including erythema nodosum (EN), Cogan's syndrome, hypocomplementemic vasculitis urticarial syndrome, erythema elevatum diutinum (EED), Eales's disease, and erythema multiforme, are discussed in this chapter. Finally, a new vasculitic syndrome characterized by hypereosinophilia, small vessel vasculitis of the skin, and vasculitis of muscular arteries of the extremities is briefly presented.

ERYTHEMA NODOSUM

Definition. EN, characterized by recurrent crops of painful, erythematous, nodular lesions, is a clinical syndrome generally associated with another systemic disease such as tuberculosis, coccidioidomycosis, streptococcal infection, or sarcoidosis. However, EN of unknown cause in an otherwise healthy individual is not a rare occurrence. The histopathology is characterized by both acute and chronic inflammation of structures in the dermis and subcutaneous tissues and may include a vasculitic component.[696-699]

Pathophysiology. The etiology of EN is unknown. Evaluating the pathophysiology of this syndrome is complicated because EN as clinically defined probably represents a heterogeneous group of disease processes.[696] Both cell-mediated and immune complex–mediated disease mechanisms have been suggested in the pathogenesis of the condition. Immunoglobulin and complement can be demonstrated in vessel walls in some EN lesions.[700] The finding of mycobac-

147

terial and streptococcal antigen in biopsies of skin lesions associated with these organisms[69] supports the concept of an immune complex–mediated mechanism. In erythema nodosum leprosum, an immune complex–mediated mechanism of inflammation is more firmly established, with antibody, complement, and lepromatous antigen demonstrated in the vessel wall by immunofluorescence.[701] The differences, however, between classic EN and erythema nodosum leprosum have been reviewed,[696] and the two entities may be distinct clinical syndromes.

The evidence of abnormalities of cellular immunity in the pathogenesis is indirect. The similarity between the histopathologic picture seen in EN and that seen in delayed hypersensitivity reactions has been emphasized.[698] The finding of EN in association with diseases that produce a host cellular immune response (i.e., tuberculosis and fungal infections), as well as with diseases in which the cell-mediated response is suppressed (i.e., sarcoidosis), suggests that the cellular components of the immune response may be involved. The precise relationship of cell-mediated and immune complex–mediated mechanisms to the pathogenesis of EN is not clearly established.

Incidence and prevalence. The incidence varies greatly depending upon factors that influence the underlying systemic disease. Variables such as the time of year, which influences the frequency of streptococcal infections, or geographic considerations, such as the prevalence of coccidioidomycosis in the Southwest, will have a great impact on epidemiologic studies. Moreover, with the effective and early treatment of streptococcal and mycobacterial infections, the frequency of EN associated with these conditions may be altered. In general, the syndrome is uncommon and appears more frequently in females.[697, 699] Although described at both extremes of age, it appears to affect the young adult more commonly.

Clinical considerations. EN usually appears suddenly as a crop of erythematous, painful, nonpruritic, slightly raised lesions on the anterior surface of the lower legs. Less frequently, a single lesion or involvement of the extensor surfaces of the forearms has been noted. The lesions vary in size from 0.5 to 2.0 cm in diameter. There is a progression from a red to a darker, purple color with intermediate color changes including yellow, green, and blue. Resolution without ulceration, scarring, or permanent pigmentary changes is generally complete in 1 to 3 weeks.

In the majority of EN cases an underlying associated disease process can be identified. Of note, EN may precede other symptoms of the underlying disease. Blomgren[696] has reviewed the group of diseases associated with EN in detail. Diseases with poorly characterized abnormalities of the host immune system, such as sarcoidosis, inflammatory bowel disease, and Behçet's disease, are associated with EN. Mycobacterial infections, including tuberculosis and lepromatous leprosy, and fungal infections, including coccidioidomycosis, histoplasmosis, North American blastomycosis, and *Trichophyton* infections, may produce EN lesions. Other conditions, including streptococcal and *Yersinia* infections as well as psittacosis and cat-scratch disease, may be associated with a clinical picture of EN. Drugs including sulfonamides, bromides, iodides, and oral contraceptives have also been causally implicated. Of note, only a minority of patients with a given underlying disease process will develop EN. Less commonly, no underlying disease process can be identified in some patients.

Pathology.   The histologic lesions of EN have been described in detail and can be quite varied.[697-699] True vasculitis may be present with primarily venous involvement.[697, 699] If biopsy is performed early in the evolution of the lesions, the inflammatory infiltrate may be composed of polymorphonuclear leukocytes; a mononuclear cell pattern is more frequent later in the course of the disease. Hemorrhage, endothelial proliferation, and a pattern of perivascular cuffing are not uncommon, whereas involvement of small arteries and arterioles is less frequently described.[697] An inflammatory infiltrate around structures in the dermis and subcutaneous tissue can be seen and may yield a pattern of panniculitis, and a granulomatous reaction with giant cell formation may be seen, particularly in the older lesions.

Diagnosis and differential diagnosis.   A diagnosis can be made clinically with confirmation by biopsy. The major clinical problem with EN is in evaluating the patient for a possible associated disease process. An appropriate evaluation will depend upon the patient's clinical presentation but should include routine blood work, chest x-ray film, skin tests, appropriate cultures, and serologic studies as well as a detailed drug history.

Treatment and prognosis.   Treatment should be directed at the underlying associated disease process. For treatment of the EN itself, a wide variety of agents, including corticosteroids, potassium iodide, aspirin, indomethacin, and colchicine, have been tried with varying degrees of success.[696, 697, 702, 703] Corticosteroids appear to be the most effective agent[697] but should be used with caution in a patient who may have an underlying infectious disease. A prudent alternative would be to try a nonsteroidal anti-inflammatory agent initially. In many patients, no treatment at all for the EN itself is indicated since the clinical manifestations generally resolve spontaneously.

COGAN'S SYNDROME

Definition.   Cogan's syndrome (syndrome of nonsyphilitic interstitial keratitis and vestibuloauditory symptoms) is a disease predominantly of young adults and consists of episodes of acute interstitial keratitis and vestibuloauditory dysfunction.[704-706] The vasculitic component observed in a minority of patients with classic or typical Cogan's syndrome is predominantly an aortitis. Systemic vasculitis is rarely encountered in classic Cogan's syndrome, and this association has frequently been confused in the literature with primary vasculitic syndromes such as polyarteritis nodosa and Wegener's granulomatosis, which may manifest ocular and auditory disorders.[706]

Etiology. The cause of Cogan's syndrome is unclear. The presence of mononuclear cell infiltrates in the cornea and structures in the cochlea (reviewed in reference 706) suggests an immune-mediated mechanism. The frequent association of upper respiratory tract symptoms prior to the onset of Cogan's syndrome suggests a possible role for an infectious agent. In this regard, serology studies have indicated a possible link with *Chlamydia trachomatis* infection in certain patients with Cogan's syndrome.

Incidence and prevalence. Cogan's syndrome is a rare disease, with just over 100 well-documented cases reported in the medical literature. The mean age of onset is in the third decade, although the disease has been reported at both extremes of age. There is a slight female predominance.

Clinical considerations. The earliest symptoms of Cogan's syndrome, as previously noted, may be related to an upper respiratory tract infection. The signs and symptoms related to the interstitial keratitis and vestibuloauditory dysfunction are generally present at the same time in a given patient. The course of interstitial keratitis is characterized by an abrupt onset of symptoms, including intense photophobia, lacrimation, and eye pain, followed by gradual improvement. Vestibuloauditory dysfunction is characterized by a sudden onset of nausea, vomiting, tinnitus, vertigo, and, frequently, progressive hearing loss.[706]

An association with other systemic manifestations has been noted.[706, 707] Aortitis with subsequent development of clinically significant aortic insufficiency may occur in 10 per cent of patients with Cogan's syndrome. As mentioned earlier, the association between classic or typical Coogan's syndrome and systemic necrotizing vasculitis is less well established.[706]

Laboratory considerations. During the acute episodes of Cogan's syndrome, a mild leukocytosis and an elevated erythrocyte sedimentation rate are characteristic. Audiograms are helpful in serially evaluating hearing fluctuations in the patient. Evidence of a recent *Chlamydia trachomatis* infection may be demonstrated serologically.

Diagnosis. The diagnosis is made on clinical grounds with documentation of the interstitial keratitis and vestibuloauditory dysfunction. Diseases that can cause an interstitial keratitis, such as congenital syphilis, tuberculosis, and viral infections, should be excluded. Systemic diseases such as systemic necrotizing vasculitis, including classic PAN, Wegener's granulomatosis, and rheumatoid arthritis, can present clinically with eye and vestibuloauditory dysfunction.

Treatment and prognosis. Daily administration of high-dose corticosteroids with a subsequent taper to an alternate-day regimen appears to be the treatment of choice. The prognosis for recovery of a hearing loss is greatly improved if therapy is initiated within 2 weeks of the onset of the decreased auditory acuity. The interstitial keratitis responds to systemic and topical corticosteroid therapy, and blindness resulting from Cogan's syndrome is extremely rare. The efficacy of corticosteroids in treating fluctuations of auditory acuity later in the course of Cogan's syndrome is less well established. These fluctuations may be related to hydrops of the cochlea rather than to recurrence of an inflammatory process.[706] Corticosteroids are also indicated when the aorta is involved. Surgical replacement of the aortic valve, in the presence of compromised hemodynamic function, has been done successfully.[707] Long-term prognosis is excellent in typical Cogan's syndrome in the absence of aortic valve involvement.[706]

HYPOCOMPLEMENTEMIC VASCULITIS URTICARIAL SYNDROME

Definition. Hypocomplementemic vasculitis urticarial syndrome is a clinicopathologic entity characterized by depression of the early components of the classic complement pathway and persistent urticaria, which on biopsy demonstrates a leukocytoclastic angiitis.[708-712] It is most closely related to the hypersensitivity vasculitides described in Chapter 5.

Pathophysiology. In the majority of cases there is a selective depression of the C1q component of complement in association with a low molecular weight (7S) protein which precipitates with C1q in agarose gels.[708-712] Immune complexes have also been identified in this syndrome,[709] and immunoglobulin and complement have been demonstrated by immunofluorescence in the walls of involved cutaneous vessels.[709] Increased clearance of C1q has also been shown in patients with this disease. The precise mechanism whereby a low molecular weight (7S) protein binding to C1q produces small vessel vasculitis presenting as an urticarial eruption has not been defined.

Of note, a patient with a familial partial deficiency of C3 has been reported to develop an urticarial vasculitic syndrome.[713] This observation suggests that depletion of the early component of the classic complement cascade may be the crucial condition for the expression of urticarial vasculitis.

Incidence and prevalence. Because the syndrome has only recently been defined, its frequency in the population has not been established. Currently, fewer than 20 well-characterized cases have been published.

Clinical considerations. The primary clinical feature is a persistent urticarial eruption. The truly systemic nature of this syndrome, however, has been emphasized.[709, 712] Additional findings include severe angioedema with occasional life-threatening laryngeal edema, arthritis, arthralgia, synovitis, neurologic abnormalities, abdominal distress, and glomerulonephritis.[709, 712] Hypersensitivity to potassium iodide has also been observed in patients with hypocomplementemic vasculitis.[711]

Laboratory considerations. The characteristic complement profile pattern is a depressed C1q with near-normal C1r and C1s levels. Other complement components including C2, C3, and C4 may be depressed. Properdin factors B and D are normal.[712] Demonstration of a 7S protein that precipitates with C1q in gels is characteristic.

Diagnosis. The diagnosis of hypocomplementemic vasculitic urticarial syndrome is established in a patient with persistent urticaria when a small vessel vasculitis is seen on skin biopsy and appropriate laboratory studies show a characteristic pattern. Serologic evaluations to exclude the diagnosis of systemic lupus erythematosus are important. Evaluation of the separate early components of the classic complement pathway is necessary to exclude C3 deficiency, which can present with a similar clinical syndrome.[713]

Treatment. Long-term follow-up and evaluation are not currently available. Antihistamines, anti-inflammatory drugs, and immunosuppressive agents have been tried,[712] but therapeutic efficacy has not been established.

ERYTHEMA ELEVATUM DIUTINUM

Definition. EED is a rare chronic skin disorder characterized by persistent red, purple, and yellowish papules, plaques, and nodules, which on histologic evaluation demonstrate a leukocytoclastic venulitis and a marked dermal inflammatory infiltrate.[714]

Pathophysiology. The etiology of EED is unknown. Increased C1q binding has been observed in the serum of patients with EED, suggesting a role for immune complexes. An association with streptococcal infection has been reported, and increased reactivity to streptokinase-streptodornase skin test antigen has also been described.[715] The relationship of these observations to the pathogenesis of EED is unclear.

Incidence and prevalence. EED is a rare disease with publications limited to case reports and small series.[716]

Clinical considerations. The cutaneous lesions, though varied, tend to have a symmetric distribution on the extremities and the sacral area. The lesions (characteristically pink, red, yellow, and purple nodules and plaques) have a predilection for the skin overlying the joints and the buttocks and are not adherent to the subcutaneous tissues.[714] Resolution with atrophic wrinkled hyper- or hypopigmented areas with loss of collagen is characteristic. The presence of systemic problems such as arthritis and streptococcal infection has been emphasized.[714]

Pathology. The characteristic pattern is a leukocytoclastic small vessel vasculitis with an infiltration by polymorphonuclear leukocytes. An inflammatory infiltrate may also be present in the upper and mid-dermis.

Diagnosis. The diagnosis of EED is established by the characteristic clinical presentation and a confirmatory pattern on skin biopsy.

Treatment. Striking resolutions of the cutaneous eruptions have been noted with dapsone treatment in an oral dose of 150 to 250 mg daily in divided doses.

EALES'S DISEASE

Eales's disease is an isolated retinal vasculitis producing a syndrome of recurrent hemorrhages in the retina and vitreous.[717] The cause of this syndrome is unknown, but the disease has been associated with tuberculosis, sickle cell anemia, and systemic vasculitic syndrome. Eales's disease is more common in young adult males. An attempt should be made to identify any underlying disorder. The prognosis for vision is guarded.

ERYTHEMA MULTIFORME

Erythema multiforme is an acute inflammatory disease of the skin and mucous membranes, usually associated with an underlying systemic process such as a drug reaction or an infectious disease. The lesion is not a true vasculitis, although a perivascular pattern with extravasation of red blood cells may be seen. Generally, the disease runs a self-limited course with complete resolution.[718]

A NEW VASCULITIC SYNDROME

A vasculitic process can, rarely, be seen in the hypereosinophilic syndrome.[719] A distinct pathophysiologic entity has been defined in

three patients who were originally included in the idiopathic hypereosinophilic syndrome (Harley, J, and Fauci, AS, unpublished observation). This disease entity is characterized by a clinical presentation of chronic atopic dermatitis, lymphadenopathy, bronchospasm,
ischemia of the digits of the upper extremities, circulating immune
complexes, and persistent hypereosinophilia. Angiography of the
upper extremities demonstrated a pattern of vasculitis of the arteries
of the hands. Histologic findings for the following sites included (1)
skin: small vessel leukocytoclastic angiitis; (2) digital artery (from
amputated specimen): infiltration of the vessel wall with mononuclear
cells and marked endothelial proliferation; and (3) lymph node:
reactive pattern.

Treatment of patients with this syndrome with cyclophosphamide
resulted in dramatic resolutions of cutaneous, pulmonary, and extremity problems.

CHAPTER 15

MANAGEMENT AND TREATMENT

INTRODUCTION

Although specific therapeutic modalities have been previously discussed for each vasculitic syndrome, an overall approach to the treatment and the management of a patient with vasculitis deserves emphasis. In the first section of this chapter, a *rationale for therapy* is discussed in relationship to treatment goals. The need for a complete diagnostic evaluation prior to the making of therapeutic decisions is emphasized. In the following section, a more detailed discussion of several *specific therapeutic modalities* is presented, emphasizing corticosteroids (CS) and cytotoxic agents as well as considering other potentially useful treatment regimens.

RATIONALE FOR THERAPY

As emphasized in Chapter 3, it is important to completely evaluate a patient with vasculitis in order to determine the extent of the vasculitic process, the diagnostic categorization, and the presence or absence of an associated underlying disease. With this comprehensive information base, a rationale for therapy can be defined and a systematic approach to treatment and management made possible. One of several treatment approaches (such as the simple removal of the offending antigen when possible, treatment of an underlying disease, or treatment directed at the primary vasculitic process) may be appropriate in a given clinical situation.

Removal of the offending antigen. In vasculitic diseases associated with immune complex deposition, the disease process can

155

potentially be halted if the offending antigen can be identified and removed. The likelihood of identifying and removing an offending antigen appears to be greatest in the group of hypersensitivity vasculitides. Drugs, infectious agents, and environmental antigens such as foods should be carefully considered as sources of sensitization. If removal of the suspect antigen results in clinical improvement, a presumptive diagnosis is established and attempts should be made to avoid the offending agent in the future. Of course, if the antigen cannot be identified, an alternative treatment approach may be necessary.

Treatment of an underlying disease.   Vasculitis can be seen in association with a wide variety of underlying systemic diseases, including rheumatic diseases, lymphoreticular neoplasms, infectious diseases, inflammatory bowel disease, retroperitoneal fibrosis, primary biliary cirrhosis, Goodpasture's syndrome, and others. Frequently, the vasculitis is a minor component of the clinical picture, for example, the vasculitis resulting from tumors, subacute bacterial endocarditis, inflammatory bowel disease, or Goodpasture's syndrome. Under these circumstances, treatment of the underlying disease often results in resolution of the vasculitis. Less frequently, the vasculitic process, particularly if present in the viscera, becomes the major clinical problem within the disease complex. For example, bowel vasculitis in patients with rheumatoid arthritis can dominate the clinical picture, and specific therapy directed at the vasculitis *per se* is clearly indicated.

Treatment directed at the primary vasculitic process.   Several approaches directed at the vasculitic process itself may be taken in treating a patient with vasculitis. Potentially, interruption of any one of several steps in the cascade of events leading to the clinical expression of vasculitis could be utilized in treating this disease process. The following are various approaches that may be taken:

1. *Prevention of deposition of circulating immune complexes in the vascular bed.* Removal of immune complexes from the circulation by plasmapheresis would be one approach in which the complexes are physically removed.

2. *Suppression of the inflammatory response, which results from the deposition of immune complexes.* Agents that modulate the expression of the inflammatory response at vessel sites following immune complex deposition include nonsteroidal anti-inflammatory agents, prostaglandins, and colchicine.

3. *Modulation of the underlying immune mechanism directly involved in producing the vasculitis.* The agents most commonly used to modulate the immune response are CS and cytotoxic agents. In reality these "immunosuppressive" agents, particularly CS, also have significant anti-inflammatory activity. Modalities less commonly employed to alter the host immune response include antilymphocyte serum and lymphapheresis.

4. *Lastly, there is empirical therapy.* Agents for which the underlying therapeutic mechanism is not clearly defined have been employed on an empirical basis with varying degrees of success. Included in this group are drugs such as dapsone, levamisole, and the potassium iodides.

The duration of therapy depends largely on the underlying vasculitic process being treated. In diseases that are self-limited, brief courses of therapy designed to suppress symptoms are appropriate. In severe systemic vasculitides, such as Wegener's granulomatosis and systemic necrotizing vasculitis of the polyarteritis nodosa group, more prolonged therapy is required to induce sustained clinical remissions. For example, we are currently treating patients with Wegener's granulomatosis for a minimum of a 1-year disease-free interval prior to tapering the immunosuppressive drugs. Generally, the drugs are tapered over a 3- to 6-month period while the patient is closely followed for evidence of recurrence of disease.

The decision to treat for a 1-year disease-free period is an empirical one, based on our experience over several years with immunosuppressive therapy in patients with Wegener's granulomatosis. The precise reason that a prolonged treatment period is required to produce and maintain clinical remissions is not clearly established. A theoretical possibility is the production of a state of immune tolerance or gradual elimination of the subpopulations of cells producing the immunologically mediated reaction requires prolonged therapy. This hypothesis, although interesting, has not been substantiated.

THERAPEUTIC MODALITIES

Nonsteroidal anti-inflammatory agents. Several nonsteroidal anti-inflammatory drugs have been demonstrated to be therapeutically efficacious in certain vasculitic syndromes. Aspirin is considered the drug of choice in the treatment of mucocutaneous lymph node syndrome[660] and may also be beneficial in the treatment of erythema nodosum.[703] However, because of its effect on platelet function, aspirin should be avoided in vasculitic syndromes such as Henoch-Schönlein purpura, in which major morbidity is caused by bleeding problems. Other nonsteroidal anti-inflammatory agents, such as indomethacin, may be of limited benefit when used in patients with Behçet's syndrome[681] or erythema nodosum.[702, 703] The newer nonsteroidal anti-inflammatory agents, including other indolacetic acid derivatives (sulindac), propionic acid derivatives (ibuprofen, naproxen), and fenamates (mefenamic acid), have not been clearly shown to be effective in the treatment of vasculitic syndromes; however, experience with these agents has been limited.[720]

Other nonsteroidal drugs with major anti-inflammatory activity, such as prostaglandins and colchicine, deserve comment. Prostaglandins have major effects in the modulation of the inflammatory response. In animal models of vasculitis, prostaglandins prevent the aggregation of polymorphonuclear (PMN) leukocytes despite deposition of immune complexes.[64] The use of this class of drugs in humans is limited, but effective use in one patient with Buerger's disease has been reported.[623] Further evaluation of this class of drugs in vasculitic disease is clearly indicated.

Colchicine, an alkaloid that has clear-cut and well-documented efficacy in the treatment of gout owing to the drug's dissolution of the microtubule system in leukocytes, has also been used to treat certain vasculitic diseases. The drug may be of therapeutic benefit in some patients with Behçet's syndrome.[689, 690] Favorable responses with colchicine have also been reported in patients with cutaneous vasculitis when the drug was used chronically in daily divided doses.[721] In this regard, patients with cutaneous vasculitis who did respond to the colchicine therapy had a leukocytoclastic pattern on skin biopsy with a predominant PMN infiltrate. A single patient in the series with cryoglobulinemia and lowered levels of complement was refractory to this therapy.[721]

Corticosteroids.   A comprehensive review of the use of CS in the vasculitic syndromes is beyond the scope of this chapter, but excellent detailed reviews on the subject have been published.[722-726] Corticosteroids are composed of 21-carbon steroid molecules. Endogenously, glucocorticoids are synthesized by a series of reactions that convert cholesterol to pregnenolone with subsequent conversion to bioactive compounds such as cortisol. Seemingly small substitutions in the glucocorticoid skeleton can have major effects on the bioactivity of the glucocorticoid, but a beta-hydroxyl group at position 11 is required for significant biologic activity.

Cortisol is the major active glucocorticosteroid produced by the body. This hormone is produced primarily by the adrenal gland, which is under the control of the hypothalamic-pituitary-adrenal axis. Although readily available, cortisol is not generally used as an immunosuppressive drug because of its sodium-retaining characteristics. With the substitution of a double bond at the 1-2 position in the cortisol structure, prednisolone is produced. This glucocorticoid analogue is more potent than cortisol on a weight basis and has reduced sodium-retaining activity. Prednisone, an analogue with keto groups at the 11 position, requires bioactivation to prednisolone in the liver. Even more potent glucocorticoids with essentially no sodium-retaining activity can be produced by substitutions of a halide in the steroid skeleton. For example, with the substitution of a fluorine at position 9 and a methyl group at position 16, dexamethasone is produced.

Knowledge of the different characteristics of the various synthetic analogues of cortisol is required for the rational clinical use of CS. Prednisone, which requires beta-hydroxylation to the active metabolite in the liver, should be avoided in patients with significant liver disease; the use of a bioactive analogue such as prednisolone would be preferred. Analogues with an intermediate half-life, such as prednisone or prednisolone, should be employed, while agents such as dexamethasone with a prolonged half-life should be avoided in alternate-day drug regimens. Because of the more prolonged biologic effect of the longer-acting agents, the hypothalamic-pituitary-adrenal axis is never free of the suppressive effects even if the drug is given every other day.

Corticosteroids given in pharmacologic doses have far-reaching effects in humans. At a cellular level the steroid molecule penetrates the cell wall to bind to a high-affinity intracellular protein (reviewed in references 725 and 727). The hormone-protein complex migrates to the nucleus, where it binds with nuclear protein and modulates gene expression at the level of regulation of specific messenger ribonucleic acids. The messenger ribonucleic acids then code for proteins that are responsible for the expression of the glucocorticoid effect.

Corticosteroids have both anti-inflammatory and immunosuppressive activities, but the mechanisms by which they produce these overlapping effects have not been fully elucidated. Multiple mechanisms contribute to the overall anti-inflammatory effects seen with CS therapy (reviewed in reference 724). An increase in the number of circulating PMN leukocytes in the peripheral blood is seen with CS therapy in man. The increased number of PMN leukocytes results from an accelerated release of these cells from bone marrow pool and decreased egress of the PMN from the circulating pool to tissue sites. This delayed egress of PMN from the circulating pool and subsequent failure to reach an inflammatory site is one of the major mechanisms by which CS prevent an inflammatory response. Functional capabilities of PMN leukocytes, such as phagocytosis or bactericidal activity, are relatively unaltered by the standard therapeutic doses of CS. In contrast to the effects on PMN leukocytes, CS produce a monocytopenia as well as inhibiting monocyte chemotaxis and bactericidal activity.[728]

The mechanisms of immunosuppression produced by CS also appear to be multifactorial. The effects of CS on mononuclear cells have been extensively studied.[729-734] A single pharmacologic dose of CS in man produces a transient lymphopenia and monocytopenia by redistribution of lymphocytes and monocytes out of the circulating pool. Within the lymphocyte subpopulation, the thymus-derived (T) lymphocytes are more sensitive than the bone marrow–derived (B) lymphocytes to this lymphopenic effect. Within the population of T lymphocytes, cells bearing a Fc receptor for IgM (T_M cells) are particularly sensitive to redistribution resulting from administration of CS, whereas cells bearing Fc receptors for IgG (T_G cells) are relatively refractory to this activity.[734] CS therapy can also directly alter the functional capacities of mononuclear cells, such as response to mitogens, cell-mediated cytotoxicity, and immunoglobulin production.[729, 732, 733] The relationship of these observations to the immunosuppression produced by CS therapy requires further definition.

CS have been used in the treatment of virtually all vasculitic syndromes and remain a major therapeutic modality for many of the vasculitic syndromes. This class of drugs is an important adjuvant in the treatment of patients with systemic necrotizing vasculitis, Wegener's granulomatosis, or lymphomatoid granulomatosis. CS are particularly important during the initial induction period of immunosuppression with cytotoxic agents. The immunosuppressive activity of CS is apparent quite rapidly, in contrast to the immunosuppressive effects of low-dose chronic regimens of cytotoxic agents such as cyclophosphamide, which are generally not realized until the second week of drug therapy. For this reason, high-dose daily CS are utilized during the initial phases of immunosuppressive therapy. When the full therapeutic effect of the cytotoxic agents is apparent, the CS can generally be tapered to an alternate-day regimen and, if appropriate, discontinued altogether.

CS are the primary treatment modality in temporal arteritis,[398] and CS have been employed extensively in the hypersensitivity group of vasculitis. The responses have been variable, and, although clinical improvement can be demonstrated in certain patients, the variability of the clinical course in this group of diseases has made the accurate assessment of the efficacy of CS therapy difficult. Long-term, low-dose therapy with CS may benefit patients with Takayasu's arteritis.[454, 455, 457] In patients with Henoch-Schönlein purpura, CS suppress gastrointestinal tract and joint-related symptoms but do not appear to alter the course of the renal lesions.[245, 285, 286] CS should be avoided in mucocutaneous lymph node syndrome, since an increased incidence of coronary artery aneurysms has been associated with steroid treatment in this disease.[660]

The concept of "steroid effect" is useful when trying to understand the rationale for various CS drug regimens. Steroid effect is the degree of biologic activity in a given regimen of CS therapy. An increase in degree of immunosuppression, anti-inflammatory activity, and hypothalamic-pituitary suppression as well as risk of frequency and severity of drug-related side effects parallels an increase in steroid effect. Multiple factors, including the selection of a CS analogue, the total dose given, the frequency of administration, and the duration of therapy, contribute to the overall "steroid effect."

In general, CS analogues with greater potency per milligram also have a more prolonged biologic effect and hence a greater overall steroid effect. For example, 15 mg of dexamethasone is a relatively large pharmacologic dose, while 15 mg of cortisol is in the physiologic range.

Obviously increasing the amount of drug in a given dose will increase the steroid effect. Perhaps less obvious, yet equally important, is the relationship between frequency of drug administration and steroid effect. Within a given time period, an increase in frequency of administration of a given total amount of CS in divided doses greatly increases the steroid effect. For example, the steroid effect of 10 mg of prednisone given four times daily exceeds 40 mg of prednisone given as a daily single dose, and 40 mg of prednisone as a daily single dose exceeds 80 mg of prednisone given on an alternate-day regimen. The total daily average dose of prednisone is identical for these regimens, but the steroid effect varies greatly.

The final variable, duration of therapy, is also of major importance. High pharmacologic doses of CS are well tolerated for brief periods of time, but with prolonged therapy the risk of adverse side effects increases and eventually becomes predictable and inevitable. Pharmacologic doses of CS given as daily or even split doses are generally well tolerated for approximately 1 to 2 weeks. After this time, side effects such as hypothalamic-pituitary-adrenal axis suppression can be demonstrated. This observed pattern is one rationale for "burst" steroid therapy whenever a short course of high-dose daily steroid is given, after which the drug is rapidly tapered and discontinued.

Other CS regimens deserve further discussion. The benefits of alternate-day CS therapy have been emphasized.[735] Given properly, alternate-day steroid therapy provides significant anti-inflammatory and immunosuppressive activity while minimizing undesirable side effects such as hypothalamic-pituitary-adrenal axis suppression and increased risk of infection.[723] Only CS analogues, such as prednisone or prednisolone, should be employed on an alternate-day regimen. Administering dexamethasone every other day will *not* result in a true alternate-day regimen, because the prolonged biologic effect of this drug does not allow the hypothalamic-pituitary-adrenal axis to escape the effect of steroid on the day in which the drug is not administered. In addition, the CS should be administered as a single dose in the morning. Finally, the dose should not exceed 80 mg of prednisone or its equivalent. Higher doses may result in a more prolonged biologic effect, which carries over into the "off" day and defeats the intent of the alternate-day regimen.

Another treatment regimen involving CS is "pulse" therapy, in which a patient is given a brief course of ultra-high intravenous doses of steroids. An example of this kind of regimen would be intravenous infusion of 1 gm of methylprednisolone daily for 3 to 5 days. The first major clinical success of this kind of CS regimen has been in the suppression of renal allograft rejection.[736] Successful CS "pulse" treatments in Goodpasture's syndrome,[737] aplastic anemia,[738] and rapidly progressive glomerulonephritis[739] have been reported. The experience with "pulse" CS therapy in vasculitic syndromes is limited. Clinical improvement in two patients with poorly character- ized vasculitic syndromes has been reported with this therapeutic approach.[740] Although intravenous "pulse" CS therapy is considered relatively safe,[741, 742] side effects including sudden death have been reported with rapid (less than 30 minutes) intravenous infusion of methylprednisolone.[743, 744] "Pulse" therapy with methylprednisolone should be considered as experimental in patients with vasculitis until further information is available.

The plethora of side effects related to CS therapy have been reviewed in detail.[725, 727] The commonly occurring major problems, including hypothalamic–pituitary axis suppression, cataracts, and os- teoporosis, are directly related to the steroid effect and are predictable in patients receiving prolonged courses of daily pharmacologic doses of CS. Attempts to minimize the side effects should be made by tapering the drug to an alternate-day regimen or by determining the minimum dose that produces the desired clinical end point.

CYTOTOXIC AGENTS

Cytotoxic drugs were initially developed for use in neoplastic diseases, but because of the observed suppression of the immune system by these agents, they have been employed in a number of inflammatory diseases.[745-747] Several classes of cytotoxic agents are used, including alkylating agents such as cyclophosphamide and chlorambucil, antimetabolites such as azathioprine and 6-mercap- topurine, and folic acid antagonists such as methotrexate. Cyclophos- phamide has been the major cytotoxic drug used in the treatment of vasculitic diseases.

Cyclophosphamide. Cyclophosphamide (Cytoxan) is a bifunc- tional substituted nitrogen mustard compound, N,N-bis(β- chloroethyl)-N$^-$,O-propylene phosphoric acid ester diamide, or 2- [bis(2-chloroethyl) amino] tetrahydro-2H-1,3,2-oxazophosphorine-2- oxide, which requires activation to an alkylating metabolite by a series of enzymatic conversions in the liver.[748, 749]

The metabolism of cyclophosphamide when used in a chronic daily low-dose immunosuppressive regimen has not been studied; however, a detailed pharmacologic evaluation of this drug following intravenous infusion for neoplastic diseases has been reported. Inject- ed radiolabeled cyclophosphamide is rapidly distributed into 64 per cent of body weight. The half-life of plasma cyclophosphamide in patients without prior drug exposure was 6.5 hours, and a peak plasma alkylating activity was seen 2 to 3 hours after infusion. In patients who had received previous doses of cyclophosphamide, the plasma cyclo- phosphamide half-life was reduced and the peak plasma alkylating activity was higher, observations suggesting that the enzymes in the liver required for activation of cyclophosphamide are inducible. In addition, although both the plasma cyclophosphamide half-life and the peak plasma alkylating activity varied markedly in patients with or without prior drug exposure, the concentration time product remained relatively constant for all patients for a given cyclophosphamide dose, suggesting that changes in the rate of metabolism of cyclophosphamide to the active analogue due to either induction or inhibition of hepatic enzymes will not alter toxicity or therapeutic effect.[748]

The majority of the radiolabeled cyclophosphamide was cleared in the urine with 62 per cent of the labeled material appearing in 2 days and 68 per cent in 4 days. Less than 20 per cent of the radiolabeled cyclophosphamide was excreted unmetabolized. Negligible amounts were present in the breath or stools. These observations on the excretion of radiolabeled cyclophosphamide suggest that the kidney is the major route for clearance of the active metabolites. In the single patient studied who had compromised renal function, detectable plasma alkylating activity was present 24 hours after the drug was given, while in patients with normal renal function the plasma alkylating activity level was never detectable at 24 hours. Of note, the patient with compromised renal function experienced a more profound leukopenia than those with normal renal function, suggesting that moderate to severe renal failure may significantly alter the toxicity and therapeutic effect of a given dose of cyclophosphamide.

At a cellular level, the mechanisms of action of the activated metabolites are unclear and may involve more than one site (reviewed in reference 747). The active metabolites have been shown to cross-link with nucleic acids, interfering with a wide variety of cellular activities. In addition, certain metabolites have the ability to phosphorylate, thereby further interfering with cellular function.

Cyclophosphamide may produce an immunosuppressive effect without a substantial anti-inflammatory effect when used in chronic low-dose regimens that avoid granulocytopenia. For example, cutaneous inflammatory responses, measured by Rebuck skin window technique in patients with Wegener's granulomatosis in remission and immunosuppressed on cyclophosphamide therapy, were normal.[330]

The mechanisms of action of the active metabolites at the subcellular level whereby an immunosuppressed state is produced have not been clearly defined. Cyclophosphamide therapy alters the circulating pool of mononuclear cells, producing both monocytopenia and lymphopenia.[330] Circulating levels of both T lymphocytes and B lymphocytes are depressed in patients on cyclophosphamide therapy,[750, 751] with greater decreases (at least initially) in the number of circulating B lymphocytes.

The functional capabilities of mononuclear cells are also altered by therapy with chronic low-dose cyclophosphamide. Lymphocyte blastogenic responses to mitogens such as concanavallin A, phytohemagglutinin, and pokeweed mitogen remain relatively intact, but responses to antigens such as streptokinase-streptodornase can be suppressed.[752] Established delayed hypersensitivity responses are unaltered, but both humoral and delayed hypersensitivity responses to new antigens may be markedly suppressed.[753] *In vitro* human B lymphocyte function, determined by a pokeweed mitogen–induced immunoglobulin secretion assay, is quite sensitive to the *in vitro* effect of the active metabolites of cyclophosphamide.[754] The B cell function in patients on cyclophosphamide therapy measured by pokeweek mitogen–triggered total immunoglobulin secretion is also suppressed (Cupps, TR, Fauci, AS, unpublished observation). The importance of these observations to immunosuppression in patients has not been fully defined, but a substantial sensitivity of B cell function to the direct immunosuppressive effects of the drug is strongly suggested.

It is of interest that cyclophosphamide has been used to induce specific immunologic tolerance in a mouse model by immunization with polyinosinic-polycytidylic acid in association with cyclophosphamide treatment.[755] Animals treated in this manner failed to mount an antibody response following subsequent challenge with the same antigen. The mechanism of this tolerance is not fully defined, but it is probably a selective depletion of antigen-activated clones by the cytotoxic drug. One may speculate whether a state of immunologic tolerance has been produced in the patients with Wegener's granulomatosis and certain other vasculitides who remain in a sustained clinical remission after cessation of cyclophosphamide therapy. However, owing to the lack of an experimental animal model for these diseases, this possibility remains an interesting, but untested, hypothesis.

Among the vasculitic syndromes, cyclophosphamide is clearly the treatment of choice in Wegener's granulomatosis[9, 371, 372] and in steroid-resistant systemic necrotizing vasculitis.[118, 138] It is also important in the treatment of patients with lymphomatoid granulomatosis.[374, 388] In addition, this drug has been tried in a variety of other vasculitides such as Behçet's disease,[692] but the indications for its use are not yet clearly defined. In patients with small vessel hypersensitivity vasculitis who develop progressive dysfunction of a vital organ, such as in certain patients with mixed cryoglobulinemia[105] or Henoch-Schönlein purpura[286, 290] with progressive renal involvement, a trial of cytotoxic therapy may be indicated if corticosteroid therapy proves ineffective.

Details of the therapeutic approach in the use of cyclophosphamide as an immunosuppressive agent have been previously reviewed.[1, 327] Generally, the drug is started at 2 mg per kg orally per day. In a critically ill patient a dose of 3 to 4 mg per kg administered intravenously for the first 3 to 4 days of induction may be indicated before converting to a 2 mg per kg oral dose. Doses higher than these levels will increase the likelihood of granulocytopenia and the risk of infection without substantially improving the clinically relevant immunosuppressive effect. Generally, we use pharmacologic daily doses of CS during the initial induction period with cyclophosphamide or other cytotoxic agents in order to provide a rapid immunosuppressive effect during the time in which the cytotoxic agent has not yet achieved an immunosuppressive effect on its own. During the second week, as the immunosuppressive effect from the cyclophosphamide occurs, an expeditious consolidation of the CS to an alternate-day regimen can be initiated.

After the initial induction period, adjustments in the cyclophosphamide dose are made in accordance with circulating peripheral leukocyte counts. In general, the degree of immunosuppression is related to the total circulating leukocyte count, being modest with a leukocyte count of 5000/mm^3, moderate at a count of 4000/mm^3, and substantial at the level of 3000/mm^3. Depressing the peripheral leukocyte count below 3000/mm^3 by chronic administration of inappropriately high doses of cytotoxic agents usually results in a selective decrease in the granulocyte count without a parallel substantial increase in the degree of immunosuppression. The degree of immunosuppression is also correlated with the total lymphocyte count. A total peripheral lymphocyte count of less than 500/mm^3 is generally associated with significant immunosuppression. In comparison, the risk of infection is more closely associated with the total granulocyte count. By maintaining a granulocyte count greater than 1000 to 1500/mm^3, the risk of bacterial and opportunistic infections is minimized. The safety of this immunosuppressive regimen, with or without *alternate-day* prednisone, with regard to infectious disease complications is well established in patients with Wegener's granulomatosis.[9, 327, 330] The only documented risk of infectious disease in patients receiving chronic low-dose cyclophosphamide therapy who are not significantly neutropenic appears to be an increased incidence of varicella-zoster virus infection.[756] Although cutaneous dissemination of the varicella-zoster infection was seen in several patients, no visceral dissemination or long-term sequelae were observed.

Several additional points should be made regarding monitoring of the peripheral leukocyte count in patients on chronic cyclophosphamide therapy. Changes in the peripheral leukocyte count lag behind changes in the cyclophosphamide dose; consequently, one should not expect immediate changes in a peripheral leukocyte count after a modification of the cyclophosphamide dose. A rule of thumb is, "The leukocyte count drawn today reflects the drug given last week." Therefore, if the peripheral leukocyte count is dropping rapidly on serial daily determinations, the cyclophosphamide dose should be

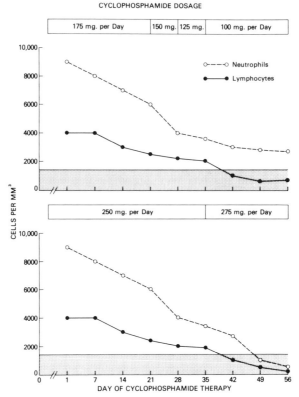

Figure 15–1. In the upper half of the figure, the neutrophil and lymphocyte cell counts in relationship to the dose of cyclophosphamide are plotted over time for a patient who is on an optimally managed immunosuppressive regimen. Note that the dose of cyclophosphamide is reduced as the leukocyte count drops, so that a suitable level of immunosuppression is obtained without suppression of the neutrophil count below 1500 cells/mm³. In the lower section, the neutrophil and lymphocyte cell counts in relationship to the dose of cyclophosphamide are plotted over time for a patient who has not received optimal management of the cytotoxic regimen. Instead of reducing the dose of cyclophosphamide as the leukocyte count dropped, the dose was increased. At this point there was a selectively greater reduction in the neutrophil count as opposed to the lymphocyte count, which had only a minimal decrease compared with the neutrophil count. The patient subsequently developed neutropenia with a total neutrophil count below 1500 cells/mm³ and was put at an increased risk of developing an opportunistic infection.

held or lowered based on this downward trend and the slope of the decline. If one waits to reach the critical neutrophil level of 1000 to 1500 cells/mm³ before altering the drug dose, the leukocyte count may continue to decline below its safe nadir, increasing the patient's risk of infection (Fig. 15–1). Frequent leukocyte counts are particularly important during the critical induction period before the individual's chronic cyclophosphamide requirement is established.

    Corticosteroids can also effect the response to cytotoxic agents. Steroids do not appear to alter the metabolism of cyclophosphamide[748] but do affect the response as measured by the peripheral leukocyte count. As previously noted, CS produce a circulating granulocytosis and lymphopenia. Patients taking pharmacologic doses of CS are *relatively* refractory to the leukopenic effects of cyclophosphamide. For a given dose of cyclophosphamide, the patient's peripheral leukocyte count generally will be higher while he is on steroids. This fact is particularly important to keep in mind following the "induction period" with cytotoxic agents, when the CS that were administered early in the induction period are being tapered. A given dose of cyclophosphamide, which produced an appropriate therapeutic decrease in leukocyte count on daily prednisone, may produce profound granulocytopenia when the patient is converted to an alternate-day CS regimen. The full effect of such manipulations of drug regimens on the leukocyte count may not be appreciated until several weeks after completion of the steroid tapering because of the lag time in drug effect, as mentioned earlier. With each alteration in the steroid dose, evaluation of the peripheral leukocyte count is needed to determine if a concomitant change will be required in the cyclophosphamide dose.

Another interesting relationship between CS administration and cyclophosphamide has been observed. Although CS can spuriously elevate the neutrophil count by mobilizing cells from the bone marrow reserves,[724] another potentially important effect of CS can be seen with regard to the concomitant administration of cyclophosphamide. It has been demonstrated in an animal model that CS "spares" the response of granulocyte precursors to the effects of granulopoietin in the face of cyclophosphamide.[375] In essence, CS can partially protect granulopoiesis from the suppressive effects of cyclophosphamide in this model. Thus, by extention to the human clinical situation, administration of CS can potentially allow the protection of granulopoiesis from the unwanted effect of the cytotoxic agent.

Because CS produce transient changes in the peripheral circulating leukocyte pool, additional care is required in evaluating patients on alternate-day prednisone. In general, the blood should be drawn before the CS is given, and baseline levels for both "on" and "off" days should be determined. The count may vary from 2500 to 4000 leukocytes/mm^3 depending upon when the blood sample is drawn. Appropriate changes in the cyclophosphamide doses can be made only if the leukocyte count is interpreted in relationship to the CS dose.

After a maintenance dose of cyclophosphamide is established, the leukocyte count remains relatively stable. Periodic checks of the leukocyte count and the platelet count are required. However, since there is a tendency for the bone marrow reserve to decline over time with chronic regimens of cytotoxic agents, a gradual reduction in the cyclophosphamide dose may be necessary.

Because there may be delayed clearance of plasma-alkylating activity in patients with renal dysfunction treated with cyclophosphamide, there is a potential for increased drug-related toxicity in these individuals.[748] Thus, the safe use of this drug requires additional consideration in the case of patients with altered renal function. The clinical situation may be particularly complex in the treatment of patients with Wegener's granulomatosis, in which relatively rapid changes in renal function can be observed. With significant compromise of renal function (creatinine clearance below 30 ml per minute), a lower dose of drug may be required to produce a given drop in the leukocyte count. Again, the leukocyte count should be closely followed until the desired end point has been reached, keeping in mind that the renal failure may result in a more gradual build-up of active metabolites, delaying the time at which a "steady-state" level is reached. To reiterate, the critical factor under these circumstances is the careful monitoring of the leukocyte count with appropriate modifications of the drug dosage in accordance with the leukocyte count.

For chronic usage, cyclophosphamide is generally given orally as a single daily dose. The long circulating half-life and even more prolonged biologic effect make more frequent administration unnecessary. Theoretically a split-dose schedule might increase the risk of bladder problems by producing a higher concentration of active metabolites in the concentrated early morning urine.

"Pulse" intravenous cyclophosphamide regimens are being evaluated in patients with lupus nephritis.[757] The drug is given as an intravenous dose of 0.5 to 1 gm per m^2 body surface area every 3 months. No experience with "pulse" cytotoxic therapy in groups of patients with vasculitis has been reported.

Both immediate and long-term complications have been reported with the use of cyclophosphamide.[745, 746] A knowledge of the associated complications is required to minimize, whenever possible, the risks to the patient. A direct effect of the cytotoxic activity of the drug is bone marrow suppression. As outlined previously, frequent and careful attention to peripheral leukocyte counts is required to avoid suppressing the bone marrow neutrophil production below a critical level at which the risk of infection is increased. In patients who continue to require immunosuppressive therapy and who have a low bone marrow reserve, the addition of alternate-day prednisone to the therapeutic regimen may allow the safe use of an increased dose of cyclophosphamide, as mentioned earlier (Fauci, AS, unpublished observations).

Complications of the lower urinary tract, particularly hemorrhagic cystitis and bladder fibrosis, have been noted. This localized complication most likely results from the active metabolites that are present in the urine. The incidence of these complications has not been well defined for patients on an immunosuppressive regimen of cyclophosphamide. In one series, 7 of 54 patients on an immunosuppressive regimen developed sterile hemorrhagic cystitis during a 241 patient-year follow-up.[758] In patients treated for neoplastic disease, the frequency and the severity of bladder fibrosis were directly correlated to the total dose of cyclophosphamide given.[759]

It is generally felt that the bladder complications can be prevented, or at least minimized, by maintenance of adequate hydration with a good urinary output.[760, 761] In this regard we attempt to maintain a daily 3-liter urine output. It is important to avoid a concentrated morning urine in order that the bladder mucosa is not subjected to increased concentrations of active metabolites. Drinking several glasses of water prior to retiring, voiding before retiring, and voiding early in the morning are recommended.

Patients with bladder dysfunction that prevents complete emptying of the bladder may be at greater risk for developing these complications. A history suggestive of urinary tract obstruction such as frequency, hesitancy, and nocturia should be thoroughly evaluated. Bladder dysfunction may be unrelated to the underlying disease process or may result from a central or peripheral neurogenic dysfunction caused by the underlying vasculitic disease process. This latter possibility should be considered, particularly in patients with isolated central nervous system vasculitis or systemic necrotizing vasculitis.

If a bladder complication occurs, the cyclophosphamide should be withheld while the problem is evaluated. Appropriate urine cultures should be done to rule out infection. Evaluation to exclude predisposing factors such as obstruction or neurogenic bladder dysfunction may be appropriate. Cystoscopy may be useful in evaluating the degree of bladder mucosal involvement. If only minimal erythema and telangiectasia are present, reinitiation of cyclophosphamide therapy with more aggressive hydration may be considered if a pressing clinical indication for the drug remains. If the cystoscopic evaluation demonstrates a diffusely hemorrhagic bladder mucosa with multiple telangiectasia and evidence of early fibrosis, the cyclophosphamide must be discontinued and an alternative cytotoxic agent considered.

Gonadal dysfunction is another major complication of cyclophosphamide therapy.[762] Incidence figures and long-term follow-ups of gonadal suppression are not readily available for patients treated with chronic immunosuppressive regimens. Premature ovarian failure is a well-established complication of cyclophosphamide therapy,[763, 764] and the incidence seems to increase with age.[765] Return of ovarian function may be seen in younger women after the drug is stopped. Histologic evaluation of the ovary may show arrested follicular maturation or absence of ova.[762, 766] The teratogenic potential of chronic cytotoxic drug regimens has not been well defined.

In males, azoospermia is frequently seen with long-term immunosuppressive regimens of cyclophosphamide.[767] The long-term risks of teratogenesis and sterility have not been defined. The use of a sperm bank for future conception is an alternative to consider for a young male who is about to be treated with cytotoxic agents.

Although the exact risk has not been clearly defined, carcinogenesis is another potential long-term complication of cyclophosphamide therapy. In a series of 54 patients with systemic lupus erythematosus or rheumatoid arthritis treated with cyclophosphamide, two cases of transitional cell carcinoma of the bladder were identified during a 241 patient-year follow-up.[758] In comparison, no cases of cancer have been diagnosed in a series of 70 patients with Wegener's granulomatosis treated with cyclophosphamide despite a 255 patient-year follow-up (Fauci AS, unpublished observations). Although the reason for the discrepancy is unclear, it may represent differences in the underlying diseases or variations in administration of the drug. Initial observations suggesting an increased risk of myelogenous leukemia in patients with rheumatic diseases treated with cytotoxic agents[768] will require further evaluation.

Other problems include gastrointestinal tract symptoms such as nausea and vomiting. Generally, this problem resolves with continued drug administration. If the nausea persists, administration of the drug in the evening may allow the patient to "sleep through" the period when the symptoms are greatest. However, care must be taken to maintain good hydration with a dilute urine if the cyclophosphamide is given in the evening. Alternatively, a brief course of intravenous drug administration may allow the patient to be restarted on an oral regimen with reduced symptoms.

Noticeable hair loss is seen in the majority of patients under chronic cyclophosphamide regimens, but generally the hair regrows despite continued therapy. However, in a minority of patients the hair will not regrow until after the drug is discontinued.

There appears to be a small but definite risk of developing pulmonary fibrosis as the result of cyclophosphamide therapy.[769] The complication may be delayed, appearing several years after completion of the drug therapy.

Chlorambucil. Chlorambucil is another alkylating agent that has been used as an immunosuppressive drug. It apparently is effective in the limited form of Wegener's granulomatosis.[326, 373] Although the spectrum of complications and side effects are similar to those of cyclophosphamide, chlorambucil does not appear to produce major problems in the bladder. For this reason, chlorambucil should be considered as an alternative agent in patients with cyclophosphamide-induced hemorrhagic cystitis who require further immunosuppressive therapy.

Azathioprine and 6-mercaptopurine. Azathioprine is the imidazole derivative of 6-mercaptopurine. Both drugs are purine analogues that act by blocking the interconversion of nucleotides, thereby affecting the synthesis of nucleic acids as well as other intracellular biochemical processes.[745, 746] Differences in the immunosuppressive

effects of cyclophosphamide and 6-mercaptopurine have been identified in animal models.[770] This class of drug is clearly not as effective
as cyclophosphamide in inducing remissions in Wegener's granulomatosis[9, 371] or systemic necrotizing vasculitis.[118] Once a patient
with vasculitis is put into remission, however, the purine analogues
may be effective in maintaining the remission in certain cases. These
drugs are suitable alternative cytotoxic agents for patients in whom
remissions have been induced with cyclophosphamide but who have
developed unacceptable complications from the cyclophosphamide
therapy. In addition to bone marrow suppression, hepatotoxicity may
be seen with azathioprine or 6-mercaptopurine.

Methotrexate. Methotrexate is a folic acid antagonist that blocks
one-carbon fragment transfers required for cellular synthesis of
purines, pyrimidines, and amino acids.[745] This activity consequently
affects nucleic acid and protein synthesis. The limiting toxicity of this
drug when used as an immunosuppressive agent is the development
of hepatic fibrosis.[746] Little information is available concerning the use
of this drug in vasculitic syndromes.

MISCELLANEOUS THERAPEUTIC MODALITIES

Plasmapheresis. Plasmapheresis involves removing substantial
volumes of a patient's intravascular fluid compartment and replacing
the fluid with a suitable colloid. This technique has been used to
remove apparently pathogenic circulating agents, such as autoan-
tibodies or immune complexes. In patients with Goodpasture's syndrome, favorable responses have been reported with plasmapheresis
combined with immunosuppressive therapy.[771-774] Clinical improvements in systemic lupus erythematosus,[775] rheumatoid arthritis,[776] and
rheumatoid arthritis with cutaneous vasculitis[777] have also been noted
following plasmapheresis. However, sustained improvement requires
the simultaneous use of an immunosuppressive agent.

The mechanism of action in plasmapheresis is not clear. Initially,
reductions in immune complex levels[775-777] and rheumatoid factor[776, 777] are observed, but a rebound to pretreatment levels, despite
continued plasmapheresis and immunosuppressive therapy, is characteristic.[776] Transient reversal of the impaired splenic component of
reticuloendothelial cell function, as measured by the clearance of
antibody-coated and heat-damaged erythrocytes, has also been reported following plasmapheresis.[40] The importance of this observation in
relation to the clinical response is not clear.

The experience with plasmapheresis in patients with vasculitic
syndromes is limited. In addition to individuals with rheumatoid
arthritis and vasculitis,[777] patients with uncomplicated cutaneous
vasculitis associated with circulating immune complexes have experienced transient clinical remissions following plasmapheresis.[40] Recurrence of the vasculitides was associated with increasing titers of

immune complexes. Consequently, chronic intermittent plasma-pheresis treatments were required for maintenance of the clinical remission.[40] Potential complications of plasmapheresis include (1) protein depletion, (2) depletion of clotting factors with increased bleeding in patients replaced with nonplasma colloids, and (3) risk of infection such as hepatitis in patients replaced with plasma. Although no systematic review of the risks of plasmapheresis is currently available, the procedure appears to be relatively safe. Certain features of plasmapheresis are prohibitive, such as the absolute requirement for good vascular access, time consumption and patient inconven-ience, and expense. Nonetheless, further consideration of plasma-pheresis as a therapeutic modality in patients with immune complex–mediated vasculitis seems warranted.

Lymphapheresis.   Induction of immunosuppression by physical-ly removing lymphocytes from the peripheral circulating pool has been attempted in patients with rheumatoid arthritis. A preliminary report has indicated limited success with this procedure.[778] No experi-ence with lymphapheresis has been reported in patients with vasculi-tic diseases, nor has induction of immunosuppression with *antilym-phocyte serum* been systematically evaluated in patients with vasculitis.

Other therapeutic modalities.   Certain other drugs may be clini-cally useful in specific vasculitic syndromes. *Dapsone* is remarkably effective in patients with erythema elevatum diutinum.[712] *Penicil-lamine*[302] or *epsilon aminocaproic acid*[303] may be of theoretical value in patients with cryoglobulinemia. *Transfer factor,*[687] *phenformin and ethylestrenol,*[688] and *levamisole*[691] may benefit selected patients with Behçet's syndrome. Administration of a *saturated solution of potassi-um iodide* may benefit certain patients with erythema nodosum.[702] *Antihistamines* may provide symptomatic relief in patients with an urticarial component to their cutaneous vasculitis.

SUMMARY

Effective treatment of a patient with vasculitis requires a com-plete systematic evaluation. Appropriate studies should be initiated to (1) establish the precise diagnostic category within the vasculitic syndromes, (2) evaluate the extent of the disease involvement (local versus systemic), and (3) exclude other treatable systemic diseases associated with a vasculitic manifestation. With this information available, a rational approach to therapy can be outlined. Depending upon the clinical setting, removal of an offending antigen, treatment of an associated underlying disease, or therapy directed at the vasculi-tic process *per se* may be appropriate. A wide variety of therapeutic modalities are available to treat a primary vasculitic syndrome, and knowledge of their use, limitations, and complications is crucial in the effective management of a patient with vasculitis.

REFERENCES

1. Fauci AS, Haynes BF, Katz P: The spectrum of vasculitis. Clinical, pathologic, immunologic, and therapeutic considerations. Ann Intern Med 89:660, 1978.
2. Kussmaul A, Maier K: Über eine bischer nicht beschreibene eigenthümliche Arterienerkrankung (Periarteritis nodosa), die mit Morbus Brightii und rapid fortschreitender allgemeiner Muskellähmung einhergeht. Dtsch Arch Klin Med 1:484, 1866.
3. Churg J, Strauss L: Allergic granulomatosis, allergic angiitis, and periarteritis nodosa. Am J Pathol 27:277, 1951.
4. Zeek PM: Periarteritis nodosa and other forms of necrotizing angiitis. N Engl J Med 248:764, 1953.
5. Zeek PM, Smith CC, Weeter JC: Studies on periarteritis nodosa. III. The differentiation between the vascular lesions of periarteritis nodosa and of hypersensitivity. Am J Pathol 24:889, 1948.
6. Klinger H: Grenzformen der periarteritis nodosa. Frankfurt Z Pathol 42:455, 1931.
7. Wegener F: Über generalisierte, septische Gefässerkrankungen. Verh Dtsch Ges Pathol 29:202, 1936.
8. Wegener F: Über eine eigenartige rhinogene Granulomatose mit besonderer Beterligung des Arteriensystems und der Nieren. Beitr Pathol 102:36, 1939.
9. Fauci AS, Wolff SM: Wegener's granulomatosis: studies in eighteen patients and a review of the literature. Medicine 52:535, 1973.
10. Carrington CB, Liebow AA: Limited forms of angiitis and granulomatosis of Wegener's type. Am J Med 41:497, 1966.
11. Liebow AS, Carrington CRB, Friedman PJ: Lymphomatoid granulomatosis. Hum Pathol 3:457, 1972.
12. Hutchinson J: Diseases of the arteries. On a peculiar form of thrombotic arteries of the aged which is sometimes productive of gangrene. Arch Surg (Lond) 1:323, 1890.
13. Takayasu M: A case with peculiar changes of the central retinal vessels. Acta Soc Ophthalmol Jpn 12:554, 1908 (in Japanese).
14. Horton BT, Magath TB, Brown GE: An undescribed form of arteritis of the temporal vessels. Mayo Clin Proc 7:700, 1932.
15. Cochrane CG, Weigle WO: The cutaneous reaction to soluble antigen-antibody complexes. A comparison with the Arthus phenomenon. J Exp Med 108:591, 1958.
16. Dixon FJ, Vazquez JJ, Weigle WO, Cochrane CG: Pathogenesis of serum sickness. Arch Pathol 65:18, 1958.
17. Cochrane CG, Koffler D: Immune complex disease in experimental animals and man. Adv Immunol 16:185, 1973.
18. McCluskey RT, Benacerraf B: Localization of colloidal substances in vascular endothelium. A mechanism of tissue damage. II. Experimental serum sickness with acute glomerulonephritis induced passively in mice by antigen-antibody complexes in antigen excess. Am J Pathol 35:275, 1959.
19. McCluskey RT, Benacerraf B, Potter JL, Miller F: The pathologic effects of intravenously administered soluble antigen-antibody complexes. I. Passive serum sickness in mice. J Exp Med 111:181, 1960.
20. Cochrane CG, Hawkins D: Studies on circulating immune complexes. III. Factors governing the ability of circulating complexes to localize in blood vessels. J Exp Med 127:137, 1968.
21. Ishizaka K, Ishizaka T, Campbell DH: The biological activity of soluble antigen-antibody complexes. II. Physical properties of soluble complexes having skin-irritating activity. J Exp Med 109:127, 1959.
22. Ishizaka K, Ishizaka T, Campbell DH: Biologic activity of soluble antigen-antibody complexes. III. Various antigen-antibody systems and the probable role of complement. J Immunol 83:105, 1959.

23. Cochrane CG: Studies on the localization of circulating antigen-antibody complexes and other macromolecules in vessels. I. Structural studies. J Exp Med 118:489, 1963.

24. Cochrane CG: Studies on the localization of circulating antigen-antibody complexes and other macromolecules in vessels. II. Pathogenetic and pharmacodynamic studies. J Exp Med 118:503, 1963.

25. Kniker WT, Cochrane CG: The localization of circulating immune complexes in experimental serum sickness. The role of vasoactive amines and hydrodynamic forces. J Exp Med 127:119, 1968.

26. Benacerraf B, McCluskey RT, Patras D: Localization of colloidal substances in vascular endothelium. A mechanism of tissue damage. I. Factors causing the pathologic deposition of colloidal carbon. Am J Pathol 35:75, 1959.

27. Cochrane CG: Mechanisms involved in the deposition of immune complexes in tissues. J Exp Med 134:75S, 1971.

28. Gocke DJ, Osler AG: In vitro damage of rabbit platelets by an unrelated antigen-antibody reaction. I. General characteristics of the reaction. J Immunol 94:236, 1965.

29. Gocke DJ: In vitro damage of rabbit platelets by an unrelated antigen-antibody reaction. II. Studies of the plasma requirement. J Immunol 94:247, 1965.

30. Henson PM, Cochrane CG: Immunological induction of increased vascular permeability. II. Two mechanisms of histamine release from rabbit platelets involving complement. J Exp Med 129:167, 1969.

31. Henson PM: Mechanisms of release of constituents from rabbit platelets by antigen-antibody complexes and complement. II. Interaction of platelets with neutrophils. J Immunol 105:490, 1970.

32. Benveniste J, Henson PM, Cochrane CG: Leukocyte-dependent histamine release from rabbit platelets. The role of IgE, basophils, and a platelet-activating factor. J Exp Med 136:1356, 1972.

33. Smyth CJ, Gum OB: Vasculitis, mast cells and the collagen diseases. Arthritis Rheum 4:1, 1961.

34. Fisher ER, Bark J: Effect of hypertension on vascular and other lesions of serum sickness. Am J Pathol 39:665, 1961.

35. Benacerraf B, Sebestyen M, Cooper NS: The clearance of antigen antibody complexes from the blood by the reticulo-endothelial system. J Immunol 82:131, 1959.

36. Haakenstad AO, Mannik M: Saturation of the reticuloendothelial system with soluble immune complexes. J Immunol 112:1939, 1974.

37. Salky NK, Mills D, DiLuzio NR, Oppenheim MS: Activity of the reticuloendothelial system in diseases of altered immunity. J Lab Clin Med 66:952, 1965.

38. Frank MM, Hamburger MI, Lawley TJ, Kimberly RP, Plotz PH: Defective reticuloendothelial system Fc-receptor function in systemic lupus erythematosus. N Engl J Med 300:518, 1979.

39. Hamburger MI, Moutsopoulos HM, Lawley TJ, Frank MM: Sjögren's syndrome: a defect in reticuloendothelial system Fc-receptor–specific clearance. Ann Intern Med 91:534, 1979.

40. Lockwood CM, Worlledge S, Nicholas A, Cotton C, Peters DK: Reversal of impaired splenic function in patients with nephritis or vasculitis (or both) by plasma exchange. N Engl J Med 300:524, 1979.

41. Henson PM, Cochrane CG: Acute immune complex disease in rabbits. The role of complement and of a leukocyte-dependent release of vasoactive amines from platelets. J Exp Med 133:554, 1971.

42. Ishizaka T, Ishizaka K, Borsos T: Biological activity of aggregated γ-globulin. IV. Mechanism of complement fixation. J Immunol 87:433, 1961.

43. Lay WH, Nussenzweig V: Receptors for complement on leukocytes. J Exp Med 128:991, 1968.

44. Henson PM: The adherence of leukocytes and platelets induced by fixed IgG antibody or complement. Immunology 16:107, 1969.

45. Cochrane CG: Immunologic tissue injury mediated by neutrophilic leukocytes. Adv Immunol 9:97, 1968.

46. Vallota EH, Müller-Eberhard HJ: Formation of C3a and C5a anaphylatoxins in whole human serum after inhibition of the anaphylatoxin inactivator. J Exp Med 137:1109, 1973.

47. Fernandez HN, Henson PM, Otani A, Hugli TE: Chemotactic response to human C3a and C5a anaphylatoxins. I. Evaluation of C3a and C5a leukotaxis in vitro and under simulated in vivo conditions. J Immunol 120:109, 1978.

48. Humphrey JH: The mechanism of Arthus reactions. I. The role of polymorphonuclear leukocytes and other factors in reversed passive Arthus reactions in rabbits. Br J Exp Pathol 35:268, 1955.

49. Humphrey JH: The mechanism of Arthus reactions. II. The role of polymorphonuclear leukocytes and platelets in reversed passive reactions in the guinea-pig. Br J Exp Pathol 36:283, 1955.

50. Cochrane CG, Weigle WO, Dixon FJ: The role of polymorphonuclear leukocytes in the initiation and cessation of the Arthus vasculitis. J Exp Med 110:481, 1959.

51. Kniker WT, Cochrane CG: Pathogenic factors in vascular lesions of experimental serum sickness. J Exp Med 122:83, 1965.

52. Cochrane CG, Aiken BS: Polymorphonuclear leukocytes in immunologic reactions. The destruction of vascular basement membrane in vivo and in vitro. J Exp Med 124:733, 1966.

53. Janoff A, Zeligs JD: Vascular injury and lysis of basement membrane in vitro by neutral protease of human leukocytes. Science 161:702, 1968.

54. Lazarus GS, Brown RS, Daniels JR, Fullmer HM: Human granulocyte collagenase. Science 159:1483, 1968.

55. Janoff A, Scherer J: Mediators of inflammation in leukocyte lysosomes. IX. Elastinolytic activity in granules of human polymorphonuclear leukocytes. J Exp Med 128:1137, 1968.

56. Weksler BB, Goldstein IM: Prostaglandins: interactions with platelets and polymorphonuclear leukocytes in hemostasis and inflammation. Am J Med 68:419, 1980.

57. Kadowitz PJ, Joiner PD, Hyman AL: Physiological and pharmacological roles of prostaglandins. Annu Rev Pharmacol 15:285, 1975.

58. Moncada S, Gryglewski R, Bunting S, Vane JR: An enzyme isolated from arteries transforms prostaglandin endoperoxides to an unstable substance that inhibits platelet aggregation. Nature 263:663, 1976.

59. Moncada S, Higgs EA, Vane JR: Human arterial and venous tissues generate prostacyclin (Prostaglandin X), a potent inhibitor of platelet aggregation. Lancet 1:18, 1977.

60. Turner SR, Tainer JA, Lynn WS: Biogenesis of chemotactic molecules by the arachidonate lipoxygenase system of platelets. Nature 257:680, 1975.

61. Goetzl EJ, Gorman RR: Chemotactic and chemokinetic stimulation of human eosinophil and neutrophil polymorphonuclear leukocytes by 12-L-hydroxy-5,8,10-heptadecatrienoic acid (HHT). J Immunol 120:526, 1978.

62. Weksler B, Knapp J, Jaffe E: Prostacyclin (PGI₂) synthesized by cultured endothelial cells modulates polymorphonuclear leukocyte function. Blood 50(Suppl):287, 1977.

63. Goldstein IM, Malmsten CL, Kindahl H, Kaplan HB, Rådmark O, Samuelsson B, et al: Thromboxane generation by human peripheral blood polymorphonuclear leukocytes. J Exp Med 148:787, 1978.

64. Kunkel SL, Thrall RS, Kunkel RG, McCormick JR, Ward PA, Zurier RB: Suppression of immune complex vasculitis in rats by prostaglandin. J Clin Invest 64:1525, 1979.

65. Sergent JS, Lockshin MD, Christin CL, Gocke DJ: Vasculitis with hepatitis B antigenemia: long-term observations in nine patients. Medicine 55:1, 1976.

66. Levo Y, Gorevic PD, Kassab HJ, Zucker-Franklin D, Franklin EC: Association between hepatitis B virus and essential mixed cryoglobulinemia. N Engl J Med 296:1501, 1977.

67. Gocke DJ, Hsu K, Morgan C, Bombardieri S, Lockshin M, Christian CL: Vasculitis in association with Australia antigen. J Exp Med 134:330S, 1971.

68. Parish WE, Rhodes EL: Bacterial antigens and aggregated gamma globulin in the lesions of nodular vasculitis. Br J Dermatol 79:131, 1967.

69. Parish WE: Studies on vasculitis. I. Immunoglobulins, βIC, C-reactive protein, and bacterial antigens in cutaneous vasculitis lesions. Clin Allergy 1:97, 1971.
70. Glass D, Soter NA, Schur PH: Rheumatoid vasculitis. Arthritis Rheum 19:950, 1976.
71. Parish WE: Studies on vasculitis. III. Decreased formation of antibody to M protein, group A polysaccharide and to some exotoxins, in persons with cutaneous vasculitis after streptococcal infection. Clin Allergy 1:295, 1971.
72. Epstein WL: Granulomatous hypersensitivity. Prog Allergy 11:36, 1967.
73. Soter WA, Mihm MC, Gigli I, Dvorak HF, Austen KA: Two distinct cellular patterns in cutaneous necrotizing angiitis. J Invest Dermatol 66:344, 1976.
74. Fauci AS, Wolff SM: Wegener's granulomatosis and related diseases. Disease-a-Month 23(7):1, 1977.
75. Pearson GR: In vitro and in vivo investigations on antibody-dependent cellular cytotoxicity. Curr Top Microbiol Immunol 80:65, 1978.
76. Herberman RB, Djeu JY, Kay HD, Ortaldo JR, Riccardi C, Bonnard GD, et al: Natural killer cells: characteristics and regulation of activity. Immunol Rev 44:43, 1979.
77. Briggs WA, Johnson JP, Teichman S, Yeager HC, Wilson CB: Antiglomerular basement membrane antibody mediated glomerulonephritis and Goodpasture's syndrome. Medicine 58:348, 1979.
78. Piomelli S, Stefanini M, Mele RH: Antigenicity of human vascular endothelium: lack of relationship to the pathogenesis of vasculitis. J Lab Clin Med 54:241, 1959.
79. Cochrane CG: Mediators of immunologically induced vascular permeability. Fed Proc 24:368, 1965 (abstract).
80. Stefanini M, Mednicoff IB: Demonstration of antivessel agents in serum of patients with anaphylactoid purpura and periarteritis nodosa. J Clin Invest 33:967, 1954 (abstract).
81. Fabius AJM: Failure to demonstrate precipitating antibodies against vessel extracts in patients with vascular disorders. Vox Sang 4:247, 1959.
82. Paronetto F, Strauss L: Immunocytochemical observations in periarteritis nodosa. Ann Intern Med 56:289, 1962.
83. Fauci AS, Ballieux R (eds): Antibody Production In Man. In Vitro Synthesis and Clinical Implications. New York, Academic Press, 1979.
84. Fauci AS, Steinberg AD, Haynes BF, Whalen G: Immunoregulatory aberrations in systemic lupus erythematosus. J Immunol 121:1473, 1978.
85. Cline MJ, Lehrer RI, Territo MC, Golde DW: Monocytes and macrophages: functions and diseases. Ann Intern Med 88:78, 1978.
86. Territo MC, Cline MJ: Mononuclear phagocyte proliferation, maturation and function. Clin Haematol 4:685, 1975.
87. Fauci AS, Stevenson HC, Whalen G, Andrysiak P: Monocyte–T cell interactions in the immunoregulation of human B cell reactivity. Clin Res 28:502A, 1980.
88. Möller G (ed): Role of macrophages in the immune response. Immunol Rev 40:1, 1978.
89. Katz P, Alling DW, Haynes BF, Fauci AS: Association of Wegener's granulomatosis with HLA-B8. Clin Immunol Immunopathol 14:268, 1979.
90. Trygstad CW, Stiehm ER: Elevated serum IgA globulin in anaphylactoid purpura. Pediatrics 47:1023, 1971.
91. Chumbley LC, Harrison EG, DeRemee RA: Allergic granulomatosis and angiitis (Churg-Strauss syndrome). Report and analysis of 30 cases. Mayo Clin Proc 52:477, 1977.
92. Patterson R, Fink JN, Pruzansky JJ, Reed C, Roberts M, Slavin R, et al: Serum immunoglobulin levels in pulmonary allergic aspergillosis and certain other lung diseases, with special reference to immunoglobulin E. Am J Med 54:16, 1973.
93. Conn DL, Gleich GJ, DeRemee RA, McDonald TJ: Raised serum immunoglobulin E in Wegener's granulomatosis. Ann Rheum Dis 35:377, 1976.
94. DeRemee RA, McDonald TJ, Harrison EG Jr, Coles DT: Wegener's granulomatosis. Anatomic correlates, a proposed classification. Mayo Clin Proc 51:777, 1975.
95. Israel HL, Patchefsky AS, Saldana MJ: Wegener's granulomatosis, lymphomatoid

granulomatosis, and benign lymphocytic angiitis and granulomatosis of lung. Recognition and treatment. Ann Intern Med 87:691, 1977.

96. Kusakawa S, Heiner DC: Elevated levels of immunoglobulin E in the acute febrile mucocutaneous lymph node syndrome. Pediatr Res 10:108, 1976.

97. Krous HF, Clausen CR, Ray CG: Elevated immunoglobulin E in infantile polyarteritis nodosa. J Pediatr 84:841, 1974.

98. Kunkel HG, Müller-Eberhard HJ, Fudenberg HH, Tomasi TB: Gamma globulin complexes in rheumatoid arthritis and certain other conditions. J Clin Invest 40:117, 1961.

99. Kellgren JH, Ball J: Clinical significance of the rheumatoid serum factor. Br Med J 1:5121, 1959.

100. Bartfeld H: Incidence and significance of seropositive tests for rheumatoid factor in non-rheumatoid diseases. Ann Intern Med 52:1059, 1960.

101. Theofilopoulos AN, Burtonboy G, LoSpalluto JJ, Ziff M: IgM rheumatoid factor and low molecular weight IgM. An association with vasculitis. Arthritis Rheum 17:272, 1974.

102. Barnett EV, Knutson DW, Abrass CK, Chia DS, Young LS, Liebling MR: Circulating immune complexes: their immunochemistry, detection, and importance. Ann Intern Med 91:430, 1979.

103. Levinsky RJ, Barratt TM: IgA immune complexes in Henoch-Schönlein purpura. Lancet 2:1100, 1979.

104. Meltzer M, Franklin EC, Elias K, McCluskey RT, Cooper N: Cryoglobulinemia — a clinical and laboratory study. II. Cryoglobulins with rheumatoid factor activity. Am J Med 40:837, 1966.

105. Grey HM, Kohler PF: Cryoimmunoglobulins. Semin Hematol 10:87, 1973.

106. Gamble CN, Ruggles SW: The immunopathogenesis of glomerulonephritis associated with mixed cryoglobulinemia. N Engl J Med 299:81, 1978.

107. Popp JW Jr, Dienstag JL, Wands JR, Bloch KJ: Essential mixed cryoglobulinemia without evidence for hepatitis B virus infection. Ann Intern Med 92:379, 1980.

108. Travers RL, Allison DJ, Brettle RP, Hughes GRV: Polyarteritis nodosa: a clinical and angiographic analysis of 17 cases. Semin Arthritis Rheum 8:184, 1979.

109. Schneider RE, Dobbins WO III: Suction biopsy of the rectal mucosa for diagnosis of arteritis in rheumatoid arthritis and related diseases. Ann Intern Med 68:561, 1968.

110. Rose GA, Spencer H: Polyarteritis nodosa. Q J Med 26:43, 1957.

111. von Rokitansky C: Ueber einige der wichtigsten Krankheitin der Arterien. Denkscher d k Akad d Wissensch 4:49, 1852.

112. Ferrari E: Ueber Polyarteriitis acuta nodosa (sogenannte Periarteriitis nodosa) und ihre Beziehungen zur Polymyositis und Polyneuritis acuta. Beitr Pathol Anat 34:350, 1903.

113. Dickson WEC: Polyarteritis acuta nodosa and periarteritis nodosa. J Pathol Bacteriol 12:31, 1908.

114. Nuzum JW Jr, Nuzum JW Sr: Polyarteritis nodosa. Arch Intern Med 94:942, 1954.

115. Zeek PM: Periarteritis nodosa: a critical review. Am J Clin Pathol 22:777, 1952.

116. Paull R: Periarteritis nososa (panarteritis nodosa) with a report of four proven cases. Calif Med 67:309, 1947.

117. Duffy J, Lidsky MD, Sharp JT, Davis JS, Person DA, Hollinger FB, Min KW: Polyarthritis, polyarteritis and hepatitis B. Medicine 55:19, 1976.

118. Fauci AS, Katz P, Haynes BF, Wolff SM: Cyclophosphamide therapy of severe systemic necrotizing vasculitis. N Engl J Med 301:235, 1979.

119. Drüeke T, Barbanel C, Jungers P, Digeon M, Poisson M, Brivet F, et al: Hepatitis B antigen-associated periarteritis nodosa in patients undergoing long-term hemodialysis. Am J Med 68:86, 1980.

120. Nowoslawski A, Krawczyński K, Brzosko WJ, Madalínski K: Tissue localization of Australia antigen immune complexes in acute and chronic hepatitis and liver cirrhosis. Am J Pathol 68:31, 1972.

121. Wands JR, Mann E, Alpert E, Isselbacher KJ: The pathogenesis of arthritis associated with acute hepatitis-B surface antigen-positive hepatitis. J Clin Invest 55:930, 1975.

122. Blau EB, Morris RF, Yunis EJ: Polyarteritis in older children. Pediatrics 60:277, 1977.
123. Fordham CC III, Epstein FH, Huffines WD, Harrington JT: Polyarteritis and acute post-streptococcal glomerulonephritis. Ann Intern Med 61:89, 1964.
124. Sergent JS, Christian CC: Necrotizing vasculitis after acute serous otitis media. Ann Intern Med 81:195, 1974.
125. Phanuphak P, Kohler PF: Onset of polyarteritis nodosa during allergic hyposensitization treatment. Am J Med 68:479, 1980.
126. Paronetto F, Deppisch L, Tuchman LR: Lupus erythematosus with fatal hemorrhage into the liver and lesions resembling those of periarteritis nosoda and malignant hypertension. Immunocytochemical observations. Am J Med 36:948, 1964.
127. Schmid FR, Cooper NS, Ziff M, McEwen C: Arteritis in rheumatoid arthritis. Am J Med 30:56, 1961.
128. Elkon KB, Hughes GRV, Catovsky D, Clauvel JP, Dumont J, Seligmann M, et al: Hairy-cell leukemia with polyarteritis nodosa. Lancet 2:280, 1979.
129. Smith CC, Zeek PM, McGuire J: Periarteritis nodosa in experimental hypertensive rats and dogs. Am J Pathol 20:271, 1944.
130. Symmers WStC: Necrotizing pulmonary arteriopathy associated with pulmonary hypertension. J Clin Pathol 5:36, 1952.
131. Knowles HC, Zeek PM, Blankenhorn MA: Studies on necrotizing angiitis. IV. Periarteritis nodosa and hypersensitivity angiitis. Arch Intern Med 92:789, 1953.
132. Fye K: The enigma of periarteritis nodosa. West J Med 122:310, 1975.
133. Ralston DE, Kvale WF: The renal lesions of periarteritis nodosa. Mayo Clin Proc 24:18, 1949.
134. Wold LE, Baggenstoss AH: Gastro-intestinal lesions of periarteritis nodosa. Mayo Clin Proc 24:28, 1949.
135. Parker HL, Kernohan JW: The central nervous system in periarteritis nodosa. Mayo Clin Proc 24:43, 1949.
136. Lovshin LL, Kernohan JW: Peripheral neuritis in periarteritis nodosa: a clinicopathologic study. Mayo Clin Proc 24:48, 1949.
137. Frohnert PP, Sheps SG: Long-term follow-up study of periarteritis nodosa. Am J Med 43:8, 1967.
138. Leib ES, Restivo C, Paulus HE: Immunosuppressive and corticosteroid therapy of polyarteritis nodosa. Am J Med 67:941, 1979.
139. Cohen RD, Conn DL, Ilstrup DM: Clinical features, prognosis, and response to treatment in polyarteritis. Mayo Clin Proc 55:146, 1980.
140. Nightingale EJ: The gastroenterological aspects of periarteritis nodosa. Am J Gastroenterol 31:152, 1959.
141. Griffith GC, Vural IL: Polyarteritis nodosa. A correlation of clinical and postmortem findings in seventeen cases. Circulation 3:481, 1951.
142. McGrae JD Jr: Perirenal hematoma secondary to polyarteritis nodosa. Arch Intern Med 104:421, 1959.
143. Ostrum BJ, Soder PD: Periarteritis nodosa complicated by spontaneous perinephric hematoma. Roentgenographic findings in three cases and a review of the literature. Am J Roentgenol Radiat Ther Nucl Med 84:849, 1960.
144. White RH, Schambelan M: Hypertension, hyperreninemia, and secondary hyperaldosteronism in systemic necrotizing vasculitis. Ann Intern Med 92:199, 1980.
145. Bircher J, Bartholomew LG, Cain JC, Adson MA: Syndrome of intestinal arterial insufficiency ("abdominal angina"). Arch Intern Med 117:632, 1966.
146. Carron DB, Douglas AP: Steatorrhoea in vascular insufficiency of the small intestine. Five cases of polyarteritis nodosa and allied disorders. Q J Med 34:331, 1965.
147. Remigio P, Zaino E: Polyarteritis nodosa of the gallbladder. Surgery 67:427, 1970.
148. Fayemi AO, Ali M, Braun EV: Necrotizing vasculitis of the gallbladder and the appendix. Am J Gastroenterol 67:608, 1977.
149. Donnelly GH, Campbell RE: Surgical aspects of periarteritis nodosa. Arch Surg 69:533, 1954.

150. Plaut A: Asymptomatic focal arteritis of the appendix. Eighty-eight cases. Am J Pathol 27:247, 1951.
151. Lin CS, Braza F: Focal arteritis of the uterus: a case report. Mt Sinai J Med (NY) 45:402, 1978.
152. Pugh JI, Stringer P: Abdominal periarteritis nodosa. Br. J Surg 44:302, 1956.
153. Jernstrom P, Stasney J: Acute ulcerative enteritis due to polyarteritis. JAMA 148:544, 1952.
154. Wood MK, Read DR, Kraft AR, Barreta TM: A rare cause of ischemic colitis: polyarteritis nodosa. Dis Colon Rectum 22:428, 1979.
155. Rosenblum WI, Budzilovich GN, Solomon C: Periarteritis nodosa with perforation of the colon: a rare complication. Report of 2 cases. Am J Dig Dis 8:463, 1963.
156. Woods AC Jr, Parry RG, Detmer DE: Successful surgical treatment of massive abdominal hemorrhage due to periarteritis nodosa. Arch Surg 97:541, 1968.
157. Han SY, Jander P, Laws HL: Polyarteritis nodosa causing severe intestinal bleeding. Gastrointest Radiol 1:285, 1976.
158. Lyell A, Church R: The cutaneous manifestations of polyarteritis nodosa. Br J Dermatol 66:335, 1954.
159. Belisario JC: Cutaneous manifestations in polyarteritis (periarteritis) nodosa. Arch Dermatol 82:526, 1960.
160. Holsinger DR, Osmundson PJ, Edwards JE: The heart in periarteritis nodosa. Circulation 25:610, 1962.
161. James TN, Birk RE: Pathology of the cardiac conduction system in polyarteritis nodosa. Arch Intern Med 117:561, 1966.
162. Thiene G, Valente M, Rossi L: Involvement of the cardiac conducting system in panarteritis nodosa. Am Heart J 95:716, 1978.
163. Roberts FB, Fetterman GH: Polyarteritis nodosa in infancy. J Pediatr 63:519, 1963.
164. Benedict WL, Wagener HP, Hollenhorst RW, Henderson JW: The ocular manifestations of the diffuse collagen diseases. Am J Med Sci 221:211, 1951.
165. Sheehan B, Harriman DGF, Bradshaw JPP: Polyarteritis nodosa with ophthalmic and neurological complications. Arch Ophthalmol 60:537, 1958.
166. Goldstein I, Wexler D: Bilateral atrophy of the optic nerve in periarteritis nodosa. Arch Ophthalmol 18:767, 1937.
167. Goldsmith J: Periarteritis nodosa with involvement of the choroidal and retinal arteries. Am J Ophthalmol 29:435, 1946.
168. Solomon SM, Solomon JH: Bilateral central artery occlusions in polyarteritis nodosa. Ann Ophthalmol 10:567, 1978.
169. Herson RN, Sampson R: The ocular manifestations of polyarteritis nodosa. Q J Med 18:123, 1949.
170. Munro-Faure H: Necrotizing arteritis of the coronary vessels in infancy. Case report and review of the literature. Pediatrics 23:914, 1959.
171. Gillespie DN, Burke EC, Holley KE: Polyarteritis nodosa in infancy. A diagnostic enigma. Mayo Clin Proc 48:773, 1973.
172. Chamberlain JL III, Perry LW: Infantile periarteritis nodosa with coronary and branchial aneurysms: a case diagnosed during life. J Pediatr 78:1039, 1971.
173. Arkin A: A clinical and pathological study of periarteritis nodosa. A report of five cases, one histologically healed. Am J Pathol 6:401, 1930.
174. Baggenstoss AH, Shick RM, Polley HF: The effect of cortisone on the lesions of periarteritis nodosa. Am J Pathol 27:537, 1951.
175. Minick CR, Alonso DR, Rankin L: Immunologic arterial injury in atherogenesis. Prog Biochem Pharmacol 13:225, 1977.
176. Helpern M, Trubek M: Necrotizing arteritis and subacute glomerulonephritis in gonococcic endocarditis. Toxic origin of periarteritis nodosa. Arch Pathol 15:35, 1933.
177. Kaltreider HB, Talal N: The neuropathy of Sjögren's syndrome. Trigeminal nerve involvement. Ann Intern Med 70:751, 1969.
178. Banker BQ, Victor M: Dermatomyositis (systemic angiopathy) of childhood. Medicine 45:261, 1966.
179. D'Angelo WA, Fries JF, Masi AT, Shulman LE: Pathologic observations in systemic sclerosis (scleroderma). A study of fifty-eight autopsy cases and fifty-eight matched controls. Am J Med 46:428, 1969.

180. Reza MJ, Roth BE, Pops MA, Goldberg LS: Intestinal vasculitis in essential, mixed cryoglobulinemia. Ann Intern Med *81*:632, 1974.
181. Somers G, Potvleige P: Relapsing polychondritis: relation to periarteritis nodosa. Br Med J *2*:603, 1978.
182. O'Neill WM Jr, Hammer SP, Bloomer A: Giant cell arteritis with visceral angiitis. Arch Intern Med *136*:1157, 1976.
183. Papaioannou CC, Hunder GG: Vasculitis of the gallbladder in a 70-year-old man with giant cell (temporal) arteritis. J Rheumatol *6*:71, 1979.
184. Frayha RA, Abu-haidar F: Polyarteritis nodosa masquerading as temporal arteritis. J Rheumatol *6*:76, 1979.
185. Halpern M, Citron BP: Necrotizing angiitis associated with drug abuse. Am J Roentgenol Radiat Ther Nucl Med *111*:663, 1971.
186. Stafford CR, Bogdonoff BM, Green L, Spector HB: Mononeuropathy multiplex as a complication of amphetamine angiitis. Neurology *25*:570, 1975.
187. Solley GO, Winkelmann RK, Rovelstad RA: Correlation between regional enterocolitis and cutaneous polyarteritis nodosa. Two case reports and review of the literature. Gastroenterology *69*:235, 1975.
188. Ho ECK, Moss AJ: The syndrome of "mesenteric arteritis" following surgical repair of aortic coarctation. Pediatrics *49*:40, 1972.
189. Rumbaugh CL, Bergeron RT, Scanlan RL, Teal JS, Segall HD, Fang HCH, McCormick R: Cerebral vascular changes secondary to amphetamine abuse in the experimental animal. Radiology *101*:345, 1971.
190. Maxeiner SR, McDonald JR, Kirklin JW: Muscle biopsy in the diagnosis of periarteritis nodosa. An evaluation. Surg Clin North Am *32*:1225, 1952.
191. Dahl EV, Baggenstoss AH, DeWeerd JH: Testicular lesions of periarteritis nodosa, with special reference to diagnosis. Am J Med *28*:222, 1960.
192. Diaz-Perez JL, Winkelmann RK: Cutaneous periarteritis nodosa. Arch Dermatol *110*:407, 1974.
193. Fleming RJ, Stern LZ: Multiple intraparenchymal renal aneurysms in polyarteritis nodosa. Radiology *84*:100, 1965.
194. Bron KM, Strott CA, Shapiro AP: The diagnostic value of angiographic observations in polyarteritis nodosa. A case of multiple aneurysms in the visceral organs. Arch Intern Med *116*:450, 1965.
195. Bron KM, Gajaraj A: Demonstration of hepatic aneurysms in polyarteritis nodosa by arteriography. N Engl J Med *282*:1024, 1970.
196. Fauci AS, Doppmann JL, Wolff SM: Cyclophosphamide-induced remissions in advanced polyarteritis nodosa. Am J Med *64*:890, 1978.
197. Longstreth PL, Korobkin M, Palubinskas AJ: Renal microaneurysms in a patient with systemic lupus erythematosus. Radiology *113*:65, 1974.
198. Kato H, Koike S, Yamamoto M, Ito Y, Yano E: Coronary aneurysms in infants and in young children with acute febrile mucocutaneous lymph node syndrome. J Pediatr *86*:892, 1975.
199. Leonhardt ETG, Kullenberg KPG: Bilateral atrial myxomas with multiple arterial aneurysms — a syndrome mimicking polyarteritis nodosa. Am J Med *62*:792, 1977.
200. Baker SB, Robinson DR: Unusual renal manifestations of Wegener's granulomatosis. Report of two cases. Am J Med *64*:883, 1978.
201. Orbison JL: Morphology of thrombotic thrombocytopenic purpura with demonstration of aneurysms. Am J Pathol *28*:129, 1952.
202. Roach MR, Drake CG: Ruptured cerebral aneurysms caused by micro-organisms. N Engl J Med *273*:240, 1965.
203. Clark RE, McNamara TO, Palubinskas AJ: Intrarenal mycotic aneurysm detected angiographically. Br J Radiol *45*:66, 1972.
204. Halpern M, Currarino G: Vascular lesions causing hypertension in neurofibromatosis. N Engl J Med *273*:248, 1965.
205. Meyers DS, Grim CE, Keitzer WF: Fibromuscular dysplasia of the renal artery with medial dissection. A case simulating polyarteritis nodosa. Am J Med *56*:412, 1974.
206. Cochran ST, Kanter SA: Ureteric changes in polyarteritis nodosa. Br J Radiol *52*:502, 1979.
207. Reimold EW, Weinberg AG, Fink CW, Battles ND: Polyarteritis in children. Am J Dis Child *130*:534, 1976.

208. Slinger WN, Starck V: Cutaneous form of polyarteritis nodosa. Report of a case. Arch Dermatol Syph 63:461, 1951.
209. Rötstein J, Good RA: Periarteritis nodosa, limited to skin and muscle: report of a case with a discussion of the practical and theoretical implications. Arthritis Rheum 1:462, 1958.
210. Ophüls W: Periarteritis acuta nodosa. Arch Intern Med 32:870, 1923.
211. Rackemann FM, Greene JE: Periarteritis nodosa and asthma. Trans Assoc Am Physicians 54:112, 1939.
212. Wilson KS, Alexander HL: The relation of periarteritis nodosa to bronchial asthma and other forms of human hypersensitiveness. J Lab Clin Med 30:195, 1945.
213. Cooper BJ, Bacal E, Patterson R: Allergic angiitis and granulomatosis. Prolonged remission induced by combined prednisone-azathioprine therapy. Arch Intern Med 138:367, 1978.
214. Alarcón-Segovia D: The necrotizing vasculitides. A new pathogenetic classification. Med Clin North Am 61:241, 1977.
215. Winkelmann RK, Ditto WB: Cutaneous and visceral syndromes of necrotizing or "allergic" angiitis: a study of 38 cases. Medicine 43:59, 1964.
216. Cream JJ: Clinical and immunological aspects of cutaneous vasculitis. Q J Med 45:255, 1976.
217. Braverman IM, Yen A: Demonstration of immune complexes in spontaneous and histamine-induced lesions and in normal skin of patients with leukocytoclastic angiitis. J Invest Dermatol 64:105, 1975.
218. Sams WM Jr, Claman HN, Kohler PF, McIntosh RM, Small P, Mass MF: Human necrotizing vasculitis: immunoglobulins and complement in vessel walls of cutaneous lesions and normal skin. J Invest Dermatol 64:441, 1975.
219. Phanuphak P, Kohler PF, Stanford RE, Thorne EG, Claman HN: Value of skin biopsy in vasculitis. Clin Res 26:123A, 1978.
220. Sams WM Jr, Thorne EG, Small P, Mass MF, McIntosh RM, Stanford RE: Leukocytoclastic vasculitis. Arch Dermatol 112:219, 1976.
221. Parker CW: Drug allergy (3 parts). N Engl J Med 292:511, 732, 957, 1975.
222. Bamji A, Salisbury R: Cytomegalovirus and vasculitis. Br Med J 1:623, 1978.
223. Vasily DB, Tyler WB: Propylthiouracil-induced cutaneous vasculitis. Case presentation and review of the literature. JAMA 243:458, 1980.
224. Soter NA, Mihm MC Jr, Dvorak HF, Austen KF: Cutaneous necrotizing venulitis: a sequential analysis of the morphological alterations occurring after mast cell degranulation in a patient with a unique syndrome. Clin Exp Immunol 32:46, 1978.
225. Soter NA, Austen KF, Gigli I: Urticaria and arthralgias as manifestations of necrotizing angiitis (vasculitis). J Invest Dermatol 63:485, 1974.
226. Soter NA: Clinical presentations and mechanisms of necrotizing angiitis of the skin. J Invest Dermatol 67:354, 1976.
227. Soter NA: Chronic urticaria as a manifestation of necrotizing venulitis. N Engl J Med 296:1440, 1977.
228. Phanuphak P, Claman HN, Kohler PF: Urticarial vasculitis. N Engl J Med 297:948, 1977.
229. Phanuphak P, Kohler PF, Stanford RE, Schocket AL, Carr RI, Claman HN: Vasculitis in chronic urticaria. J Allergy Clin Immunol 65:436, 1980.
230. Andrews BS, Cains G, McIntosh J, Petts V, Penny R: Circulating and tissue immune complexes in cutaneous vasculitis. J Clin Lab Immunol 1:311, 1979.
231. Levine BB: Immunologic mechanisms of penicillin allergy. A haptenic model system for the study of allergic diseases of man. N Engl J Med 275:1115, 1966.
232. Han T, Chawla PL, Sokal JE: Sulfapyridine-induced serum-sickness–like syndrome associated with plasmacytosis, lymphocytosis and multiclonal gamma-globulinopathy. N Engl J Med 280:547, 1969.
233. Clark E, Kaplan BI: Endocardial arterial and other mesenchymal alterations associated with serum sickness in man. Arch Pathol 24:458, 1937.
234. MacKenzie GM, Hanger FM: Serum disease and serum accidents. JAMA 94:260, 1930.

235. Reisman RE, Rose NR, Witebsky E, Arbesman CE: Serum sickness. II. Demonstration and characteristics of antibodies. J Allergy 32:531, 1961.
236. De La Pava S, Nigogosyan G, Pickren JW: Fatal glomerulonephritis after receiving horse anti-human-cancer serum. Report of three cases. Arch Intern Med 109:67, 1962.
237. Vaughan JH, Barnett EV, Leadley PJ: Serum sickness. Evidence in man of antigen-antibody complexes and free light chains in the circulation during the acute reaction. Ann Intern Med 67:596, 1967.
238. Gilliam JN, Smiley JD: Cutaneous necrotizing vasculitis and related disorders. Ann Allergy 37:328, 1976.
239. Copeman PWM, Ryan TJ: The problems of classification of cutaneous angiitis with reference to histopathology and pathogenesis. Br J Dermatol 82(Suppl 5):2, 1970.
240. Heberden W: Commentaries on the History and Cure of Diseases. London, 1806, p. 396.
241. Willan R: On Cutaneous Diseases. London, J. Johnson, 1808.
242. Schönlein JL: Allgemeine und Specielle Pathologie und Therapie. Vol 2, 3rd ed. Herisau, Lit-Compt, 1837, p. 48.
243. Henoch E: Über eine eigenthümliche form von purpura. Berl. Klin Wochenschr 11:641, 1874.
244. Henoch E: Vorlesungen über Kinderkrankheiten, 10th ed. Berlin, A. Hirschwald, 1899, p. 839.
245. Osler W: Visceral lesions of purpura and allied conditions. Br Med J 1:517, 1914.
246. Glanzmann E: Die Konzeption der anaphylaktoiden purpura. Jahrb P Kinderh 91:391, 1920.
247. Gairdner D: The Schönlein-Henoch syndrome (anaphylactoid purpura). Q J Med 17:95, 1948.
248. Ansell BM: Henoch-Schönlein purpura with particular reference to the prognosis of the renal lesion. Br J Dermatol 82:211, 1970.
249. Cream JJ, Gumpel JM, Peachey RDG: Schönlein-Henoch purpura in the adult. A study of 77 adults with anaphylactoid or Schönlein-Henoch purpura. Q J Med 39:461, 1970.
250. Meadow SR, Glasgow EF, White RHR, Moncrieff MW, Cameron JS, Ogg CS: Schönlein-Henoch nephritis. Q J Med 41:241, 1972.
251. Allen DM, Diamond LK, Howell DA: Anaphylactoid purpura in children (Schönlein-Henoch syndrome). Review with a follow-up of the renal complications. Am J Dis Child 99:833, 1960.
252. Ballard HS, Eisinger RP, Gallo G: Renal manifestations of the Henoch-Schoenlein syndrome in adults. Am J Med 49:328, 1970.
253. Alexander HL, Eyermann CH: Food allergy in Henoch's purpura. Arch Dermatol Syph 16:322, 1927.
254. Alexander HL, Eyermann CH: Allergic purpura. JAMA 92:2092, 1929.
255. Ackroyd JF: Allergic purpura, including purpura due to foods, drugs and infections. Am J Med 14:605, 1953.
256. Jensen B: Schönlein-Henoch's purpura. Three cases with fish or penicillin as antigen. Acta Med Scand 152:61, 1955.
257. Sharan G, Anand RK, Sinha KP: Schönlein-Henoch syndrome after insect bite. Br Med J 1:656, 1966.
258. Jiménez EL, Dorrington HJ: Vaccination and Henoch-Schoenlein purpura. N Engl J Med 279:1171, 1968.
259. Casteels-van Daele M: Vaccination and Henoch-Schönlein purpura (concluded). N Engl J Med 280:781, 1969.
260. Damjanov I, Amato JA: Progression of renal disease in Henoch-Schönlein purpura after influenza vaccination. JAMA 242:2555, 1979.
261. Rogers PW, Bunn SM Jr, Kurtzman NA, White MG: Schönlein-Henoch syndrome associated with exposure to cold. Arch Intern Med 128:782, 1971.
262. Silber DL: Henoch-Schoenlein purpura. Pediatr Clin North Am 19:1061, 1972.
263. De La Faille-Kuyper EHB, Kater L, Kooiker CJ, Mees EJD: IgA-deposits in cutaneous blood vessel walls and mesangium in Henoch-Schönlein syndrome. Lancet 1:892, 1973.

264. Zuckner, J, Tsai C, Giangiacomo J, Baldassare AR, Auclair R: IgA deposition in normal and purpuric skin of patients with Henoch-Schönlein purpura. Arthritis Rheum 20:395, 1977.
265. Kuno-Sakai H, Sakai H, Nomoto Y, Takakura I, Kimura M: Increase of IgA-bearing peripheral blood lymphocytes in children with Henoch-Schoenlein purpura. Pediatrics 64:918, 1979.
266. Hyman LR, Wagnild JP, Beirne GJ, Burkholder PM: Immunoglobulin-A distribution in glomerular disease: analysis of immunofluorescence localization and pathogenetic significance. Kidney Int 3:397, 1973.
267. Evans DJ, Williams DG, Peters DK, Sissons JGP, Boulton-Jones JM, Ogg CS, et al; Glomerular deposition of properdin in Henoch-Schönlein syndrome and idiopathic focal nephritis. Br Med J 3:326, 1973.
268. Mauer SM, Sutherland DER, Howard RJ, Fish AJ, Najarian JS, Michael AF: The glomerular mesangium. III. Acute immune mesangial injury: a new model of glomerulonephritis. J Exp Med 137:553, 1973.
269. Lowance DC, Mullins JD, McPhaul JJ: Immunoglobulin A (IgA) associated glomerulonephritis. Kidney Int 3:167, 1973.
270. Lawrence DA, Weigle WO, Spiegelberg HL: Immunoglobulins cytophilic for human lymphocytes, monocytes, and neutrophils. J Clin Invest 55:368, 1975.
271. Van Epps DE, Williams RC Jr: Suppression of leukocyte chemotaxis by human IgA myeloma components. J Exp Med 144:1227, 1976.
272. Götze O, Müller-Eberhard HJ: The C3-activator system: an alternate pathway of complement activation. J Exp Med 134:90, 1971.
273. Sussman M, Jones JH, Almeida JD, Lachmann P: Deficiency of the second component of complement associated with anaphylactoid purpura and presence of mycoplasma in the serum. J Clin Exp Immunol 14:531, 1973.
274. Gelfand EW, Clarkson JE, Minta JO: Selective deficiency of the second component of complement in a patient with anaphylactoid purpura. Clin Immunol Immunopathol 4:269, 1975.
275. Feldt RH, Stickler GB: The gastrointestinal manifestations of anaphylactoid purpura in children. Proc Staff Meet Mayo Clin 37:465, 1962.
276. Garner JAMcV: Acute pancreatitis as a complication of anaphylactoid (Henoch-Schönlein) purpura. Arch Dis Child 52:971, 1977.
277. Puppala AR, Cheng JC, Steinheber FU: Pancreatitis — a rare complication of Schönlein-Henoch purpura. Am J Gastroenterol 69:101, 1978.
278. Wolfsohn H: Purpura and intussusception. Arch Dis Child 22:242, 1947.
279. Lindenauer SM, Tank ES: Surgical aspects of Henoch-Schönlein's purpura. Surgery 59:982, 1966.
280. Noussias M, Blandy AC, Ward-McQuaid N: Intussusception in Henoch-Schönlein purpura. Br J Surg 56:503, 1969.
281. Stremple JF, Polacek MA, Ellison EH: The acute nonsurgical abdomen of Henoch-Schönlein syndrome in the elderly patient. Am J Surg 115:870, 1968.
282. Imai T, Matsumoto S: Anaphylactoid purpura with cardiac involvement. Arch Dis Child 45:727, 1970.
283. Lewis IC, Philpott MG: Neurological complications in the Schönlein-Henoch syndrome. Arch Dis Child 31:369, 1956.
284. Grossman H, Berdon WE, Baker DH: Abdominal pain in Schönlein-Henoch syndrome. Its correlation with small bowel barium roentgen study. Am J Dis Child 108:67, 1964.
285. Young DG: Chronic intestinal obstruction following Henoch-Schönlein disease. Clin Pediatr 3:737, 1964.
286. Norkin S, Wiener J: Henoch-Schoenlein syndrome. Am J Clin Pathol 33:55, 1960.
287. Scully RE, Galdabini JJ, McNeely BU: Case records of the Massachusetts General Hospital (Case 14-1980). N Engl J Med 302:853, 1980.
288. Borges WH: Anaphylactoid purpura. Med Clin North Am 56:201, 1972.
289. Oliver TK, Barnett HL: The incidence and prognosis of nephritis associated with anaphylactoid (Schönlein-Henoch) purpura in children. Am J Dis Child 90:544, 1955.
290. White RHR, Cameron JS, Trounce JR: Immunosuppressive therapy in steroid-

resistant proliferative glomerulonephritis accompanied by nephrotic syndrome. Br Med J 2:853, 1966.

291. Grupe WE, Heymann W: Cytotoxic drugs in steroid-resistant renal disease. Alkylating and antimetabolic agents in the treatment of nephrotic syndrome, lupus nephritis, chronic glomerulonephritis, and purpura nephritis in children. Am J Dis Child 112:448, 1966.

292. LoSpalluto J, Dorward B, Miller W Jr, Ziff M: Cryoglobulinemia based on interaction between a gamma macroglobulin and 7S gamma globulin. Am J Med 32:142, 1962.

293. Meltzer M, Franklin EC: Cryoglobulinemia — a study of twenty-nine patients. I. IgG and IgM cryoglobulins and factors affecting cryoprecipitability. Am J Med 40:828, 1966.

294. Brouet J, Clauvel J, Danon F, Klein M, Seligmann M: Biologic and clinical significance of cryoglobulins. A report of 86 cases. Am J Med 57:775, 1974.

295. Capra JD, Winchester RJ, Kunkel HG: Hypergammaglobulinemic purpura. Studies on the unusual anti-γ-globulins characteristic of the sera of these patients. Medicine 50:125, 1971.

296. Riethmüller G, Meltzer M, Franklin E, Miescher PA: Serum complement levels in patients with mixed (IgM-IgG) cryoglobulinemia. Clin Exp Immunol 1:337, 1966.

297. Cream JJ: Cryoglobulins in vasculitis. Clin Exp Immunol 10:117, 1972.

298. Capra JD, Winchester RJ, Kunkel HG: Cold-reactive rheumatoid factors in infectious mononucleosis and other diseases. Arthritis Rheum 12:67, 1969.

299. Bombardieri S, Paoletti P, Ferri C, Di Munno O, Fornai E, Giuntini C: Lung involvement in essential mixed cryoglobulinemia. Am J Med 66:748, 1979.

300. Invernizzi F, Pioltelli P, Cattaneo R, Gavazzeni V, Borzini P, Monti G, Zanussi C: A long-term follow-up study in essential cryoglobulinemia. Acta Haemtol 61:93, 1979.

301. Capra JD: Clinical and immunologic observations in hypergammaglobulinemic purpura. Mt Sinai J Med (NY) 38:375, 1971.

302. Langlands DR, Dawkins RL, Matz LR, Cobain TJ, Goatcher P, Papadimitriou JM, et al: Arthritis associated with a crystallizing cryoprecipitable IgG paraprotein. Am J Med 68:461, 1980.

303. Lalezari P, Kumar M: Inhibition of cold insolubility of serum cryoglobulin by epsilon aminocaprioic acid. Am J Med 68:629, 1980.

304. Christian CL, Sergent SS: Vasculitis syndromes: clinical and experimental models. Am J Med 61:385, 1976.

305. Sokoloff, L, Wilens SL, Bunim JJ: Arteritis of striated muscle in rheumatoid arthritis. Am J Pathol 27:157, 1951.

306. Sokoloff, L, Bunim JJ: Vascular lesions in rheumatoid arthritis. J Chronic Dis 5:668, 1957.

307. Mongan ES, Cass RM, Jacox RF, Vaughan JH: A study of the relation of seronegative and seropositive rheumatoid arthritis to each other and to necrotizing vasculitis. Am J Med 47:23, 1969.

308. Franco AE, Schur PH: Hypocomplementemia in rheumatoid arthritis. Arthritis Rheum 14:231, 1971.

309. Weisman M, Zvaifler N: Cryoimmunoglobulinemia in rheumatoid arthritis. Significance in serum of patients with rheumatoid vasculitis. J Clin Invest 56:725, 1975.

310. Stage DE, Mannik M: 7SγM-globulin in rheumatoid arthritis: evaluation of its clinical significance. Arthritis Rheum 14:440, 1971.

311. Soter NA, Austen KF, Gigli I: The complement system in necrotizing angiitis of the skin. Analysis of complement component activities in serum of patients with concomitant collagen-vascular diseases. J Invest Dermatol 63:219, 1974.

312. Kemper JW, Baggenstoss AH, Slocumb CH: The relationship of therapy with cortisone to the incidence of vascular lesions in rheumatoid arthritis. Ann Intern Med 46:831, 1957.

313. Estes D, Christian CL: The natural history of systemic lupus erythematosus by prospective analysis. Medicine 50:85, 1971.

314. Mintz G, Fraga A: Arteritis in systemic lupus erythematosus. Arch Intern Med 116:55, 1965.

315. McCombs RP: Systemic "allergic" vasculitis. Clinical and pathological relationships. JAMA *194*:1059, 1965.
316. Sams WM Jr, Harville DD, Winkelmann RK: Necrotising vasculitis associated with lethal reticuloendothelial diseases. Br J Dermatol *80*:555, 1966.
317. Brandrup F, Østergaard PA: α_1-antitrypsin deficiency associated with persistent cutaneous vasculitis. Occurrence in a child with liver disease. Arch Dermatol *114*:921, 1978.
318. Goldman JA, Casey HL, Davidson ED, Hersh T, Pirozzi D: Vasculitis associated with intestinal bypass surgery. Arch Dermatol *115*:725, 1979.
319. Weinberger A, Myers AR: Relapsing polychondritis associated with cutaneous vasculitis. Arch Dermatol *115*:980, 1979.
320. Fahey J, Leonard E, Churg J, Godman G: Wegener's granulomatosis. Am J Med *17*:168, 1954.
321. Godman GC, Churg J: Wegener's granulomatosis. Pathology and review of the literature. Arch Pathol *58*:533, 1954.
322. Norton WL, Suki W, Strunk S: Combined corticosteroid and azathioprine therapy in two patients with Wegener's granulomatosis. Arch Intern Med *121*:554, 1968.
323. Aldo MA, Benson MD, Comerford FR, Cohen AS: Treatment of Wegener's granulomatosis with immunosuppressive agents. Description of renal ultrastructure. Arch Intern Med *126*:198, 1970.
324. Raitt JW: Wegener's granulomatosis: treatment with cytotoxic agents and adrenocorticoids. Ann Intern Med *74*:344, 1971.
325. Novack SN, Pearson CM: Cyclophosphamide therapy in Wegener's granulomatosis. N Engl J Med *284*:938, 1971.
326. Israel HL, Patchefsky AS: Wegener's granulomatosis of lung: diagnosis and treatment. Experience with 12 cases. Ann Intern Med *74*:881, 1971.
327. Wolff SM, Fauci AS, Horn RG, Dale DC: Wegener's granulomatosis. Ann Intern Med *81*:513, 1974.
328. Shillitoe EJ, Lehner T, Lessof MH, Harrison DFN: Immunological features of Wegener's granulomatosis. Lancet *1*:281, 1974.
329. Horn RG, Fauci AS, Rosenthal AS, Wolff SM: Renal biopsy pathology in Wegener's granulomatosis. Am J Pathol *74*:423, 1974.
330. Dale DC, Fauci AS, Wolff SM: The effect of cyclophosphamide on leukocyte kinetics and susceptibility to infection in patients with Wegener's granulomatosis. Arthritis Rheum *16*:657, 1973.
331. Niinaka T, Okochi T, Watanabe Y, Sakai S, Takahashi Y, Yamamura Y: Lymphocyte functions in Wegener's granulomatosis. J Med 9:491, 1978.
332. Donald KJ, Edwards RL, McEvoy JDS: An ultrastructural study of the pathogenesis of tissue injury in limited Wegener's granulomatosis. Pathology 8:161, 1976.
333. Niinaka T, Okochi T, Watanbe Y, Takahashi Y, Yamamura Y: Chemotactic defect in Wegener's granulomatosis. J Med 8:161, 1977.
334. Howell SB, Epstein WV: Circulating immunoglobulin complexes in Wegener's granulomatosis. Am J Med *60*:259, 1976.
335. Juncos LI, Alexander RW, Marbury TC: Intravascular clotting preceding crescent formation in a patient with Wegener's granulomatosis and rapidly progressive glomerulonephritis. Nephron *24*:17, 1979.
336. Walton EW: Giant-cell granuloma of the respiratory tract (Wegener's granulomatosis). Br Med J *2*:265, 1958.
337. Reed WB, Jensen AK, Konwaler BE, Hunter D: The cutaneous manifestations in Wegener's granulomatosis. Acta Derm Venereol (Stockh) *43*:250, 1963.
338. Cassan SM, Coles DT, Harrison EG: The concept of limited forms of Wegener's granulomatosis. Am J Med *49*:366, 1970.
339. Hensley MJ, Feldman NT, Lazarus JM, Galvanek EG: Diffuse pulmonary hemorrhage and rapidly progressive renal failure. An uncommon presentation of Wegener's granulomatosis. Am J Med *66*:894, 1979.
340. Haynes BF, Fishman MC, Fauci AS, Wolff SM: The ocular manifestations of Wegener's granulomatosis. Fifteen years experience and review of the literature. Am J Med *63*:131, 1977.
341. Schramm VL, Myers EN, Rogerson DR: The masquerade of vasculitis: head and neck diagnosis and management. Laryngoscope *88*:1922, 1978.

342. Fauci AS, Johnson RE, Wolff SM: Radiation therapy of midline granuloma. Ann Intern Med 84:140, 1976.
343. Morgan AD, O'Neil R: The oral complications of polyarteritis and giant-cell granulomatosis (Wegener's granulomatosis). Oral Surg 9:845, 1956.
344. Cawson RA: Gingival changes in Wegener's granulomatosis. Br Dent J 118:30, 1965.
345. Kakehashi S, Hamner JE III, Baer PN, McIntire JA: Wegener's granulomatosis. Report of a case involving the gingiva. Oral Surg 19:120, 1965.
346. Scott J, Finch LD: Wegener's granulomatosis presenting as gingivitis. Review of the clinical and pathologic features and report of a case. Oral Surg 34:920, 1972.
347. Hensle TW, Mitchell ME, Crooks KK, Robinson D: Urologic manifestations of Wegener granulomatosis. Urology 12:553, 1978.
348. Pritchard MH, Gow PJ: Wegener's granulomatosis presenting as rheumatoid arthritis (two cases). Proc R Soc Med 69:501, 1976.
349. Cupps TR, Fauci AS: Wegener's granulomatosis. Int J Dermatol 19:76, 1980.
350. DeOreo GA: Wegener's granulomatosis. Arch Dermatol 81:169, 1960.
351. Kraus Z, Vortel V, Fingerland A, Salavec M, Krch V: Unusual cutaneous manifestations in Wegener's granulomatosis. Acta Derm Venereol (Stockh) 45:288, 1965.
352. Matsuda S, Mitsukawa S, Ishii N, Shirai M: A case of Wegener's granulomatosis with necrosis of the penis. Tohoku J Exp Med 118:145, 1976.
353. Austin P, Green WR, Sallyer DC, Walsh FB, Kleinfelter HT: Peripheral corneal degeneration and occlusive vasculitis in Wegener's granulomatosis. Am J Ophthalmol 85:311, 1978.
354. Biglan AW, Brown SI, Cignetti FE, Linn JG: Corneal perforation in Wegener's granulomatosis treated with corneal transplant: case report. Ann Ophthalmol 9:799, 1977.
355. Diaz-Jouanen E, Alarcon-Segovia D: Chondritis of the ear in Wegener's granulomatosis. Arthritis Rheum 20:1286, 1977.
356. McCrea PC, Childers RW: Two unusual cases of giant cell myocarditis associated with mitral stenosis and with Wegener's syndrome. Br Heart J 26:490, 1964.
357. Levine H, Madden TJ: Wegener's granulomatosis. Report of a case. Am Heart J 53:632, 1957.
358. Drachman DA: Neurological complications of Wegener's granulomatosis. Arch Neurol 8:145, 1963.
359. Haynes BF, Fauci AS: Diabetes insipidus associated with Wegener's granulomatosis successfully treated with cyclophosphamide. N Engl J Med 299:764, 1978.
360. McGregor MB, Sandler G: Wegener's granulomatosis. A clinical and radiological survey. Br J Radiol 37:430, 1964.
361. Felson B: Less familiar roentgen patterns of pulmonary granulomas. Sarcoidosis, histoplasmosis and noninfectious necrotizing granulomatosis (Wegener's syndrome). Am J Roentgenol Radiat Ther Nucl Med 81:211, 1959.
362. Flye MW, Mundinger GH Jr, Fauci AS: Diagnostic and therapeutic aspects of the surgical approach to Wegener's granulomatosis. J Thorac Cardiovasc Surg 77:331, 1979.
363. Maguire R, Fauci AS, Doppmann JL, Wolff SM: Unusual radiographic features of Wegener's granulomatosis. Am J Roentgenol 130:233, 1978.
364. Vermess M, Haynes BF, Fauci AS, Wolff SM: Computer assisted tomography of orbital lesions in Wegener's granulomatosis. J Comput Assist Tomogr 2:45, 1978.
365. Hu C, O'Loughlin S, Winkelman RK: Cutaneous manifestations of Wegener granulomatosis. Arch Dermatol 113:175, 1977.
366. Edwards MB, Buckerfield JP: Wegener's granulomatosis: a case with primary mucocutaneous lesions. Oral Surg 46:53, 1978.
367. Goodpasture EW: The significance of certain pulmonary lesions in relation to the etiology of influenza. Am J Med Sci 158:863, 1919.
368. Lerner R, Glassock RJ, Dixon FJ: The role of antiglomerular basement membrane antibody on the pathogenesis of human glomerulonephritis. J Exp Med 126:989, 1967.

369. McPhaue JJ Jr, Dixon FJ: Characterization of human antiglomerular basement membrane antibodies eluted from glomerulonephritic kidneys. J Clin Invest 49:308, 1976.
370. Hollander D, Manning RT: The use of alkylating agents in the treatment of Wegener's granulomatosis. Ann Intern Med 67:393, 1967.
371. Reza MJ, Dornfeld L, Goldberg LS, Bluestone R, Pearson CM: Wegener's granulomatosis. Long term followup of patients treated with cyclophosphamide. Arthritis Rheum 18:501, 1975.
372. Moorthy AV, Chesney RW, Segar WE, Groshong T: Wegener granulomatosis in childhood: prolonged survival following cytotoxic therapy. J Pediatr 91:611, 1977.
373. Israel HI, Patchefsky AS: Treatment of Wegener's granulomatosis of lung. Am J Med 58:671, 1975.
374. Fauci AS: Granulomatous vasculitides: distinct but related. Ann Intern Med 87:782, 1977.
375. Joyce RA, Chervenick PA: Corticosteroid effect on granulopoiesis in mice after cyclophosphamide. J Clin Invest 60:277, 1977.
376. Eagleton LE, Rosher RB, Hawe A, Bilinsky RT: Radiation therapy and mechanical dilation of endobronchial obstruction secondary to Wegener's granulomatosis. Chest 76:609, 1979.
377. Fauci AS, Balow JE, Brown R, Chazan J, Steinman T, Sahyoun AI, et al: Successful renal transplantation in Wegener's granulomatosis. Am J Med 60:437, 1976.
378. Steinman TI, Jaffe BF, Monaco AP, Wolff SM, Fauci AS: Recurrence of Wegener's granulomatosis after kidney transplantation. Successful re-induction of remission with cyclophosphamide. Am J Med 68:458, 1980.
379. Katzenstein AA, Carrington CB, Liebow AA: Lymphomatoid granulomatosis. A clinicopathologic study of 152 cases. Cancer 43:360, 1979.
380. Hammar SP, Gortner D, Sumida S, Bockus D: Lymphomatoid granulomatosis: association with retroperitoneal fibrosis and evidence of impaired cell-mediated immunity. Am Rev Respir Dis 115:1045, 1977.
381. Kokmen E, Billman JK Jr, Abell MR: Lymphomatoid granulomatosis clinically confined to the CNS. A case report. Arch Neurol 34:782, 1977.
382. Gibbs AR: Lymphomatoid granulomatosis — a condition with affinities to Wegener's granulomatosis and lymphoma. Thorax 32:71, 1977.
383. Yockey CC, Leichter SB, Hampton JR III: Lymphomatoid granulomatosis presenting as fever of unknown origin. JAMA 237:2633, 1977.
384. Saldana MJ, Patchefsky AS, Israel HI, Atkinson GW: Pulmonary angiitis and granulomatosis. The relationship between histological features, organ involvement, and response to treatment. Hum Pathol 8:391, 1977.
385. Hammar S, Mennemeyer R: Lymphomatoid granulomatosis in a renal transplant recipient. Hum Pathol 7:111, 1976.
386. Bone RC, Vernon M, Sobonya RE, Rendon H: Lymphomatoid granulomatosis. Report of a case and review of the literature. Am J Med 65:709, 1978.
387. Peña, CE: Lymphomatoid granulomatosis with cerebral involvement. Light and electron microscopic study of a case. Acta Neuropathol (Berl) 37:193, 1977.
388. Lee SC, Roth LM, Brashear RE: Lymphomatoid granulomatosis. A clinicopathologic study of four cases. Cancer 38:846, 1976.
389. Verity MA, Wolfson WL: Cerebral lymphomatoid granulomatosis. A report of two cases, with disseminated necrotizing leukoencephalopathy in one. Acta Neuropathol (Berl) 36:117, 1976.
390. Fuller PSB, Hafermann DR, Byrd RB, Jenkins DW: Use of irradiation in lymphomatoid granulomatosis. Chest 74:105, 1978.
391. Goodman BW Jr: Temporal arteritis. Am J Med 67:839, 1979.
392. Horton BT, Magath TB: Arteritis of the temporal vessels: report of seven cases. Mayo Clinic Proc 12:548, 1937.
393. Jennings GH: Arteritis of the temporal vessels. Lancet 1:424, 1938.
394. Gilmour JR: Giant-cell chronic arteritis. J Pathol 53:263, 1941.
395. Paulley JW, Hughes JP: Giant-cell arteritis, or arteritis of the aged. Br Med J 2:1562, 1960.
396. Hauser WA, Ferguson RH, Holley KE, Kurland LT: Temporal arteritis in Rochester, Minnesota, 1951 to 1967. Mayo Clin Proc 46:597, 1971.

397. Huston KA, Hunder GG, Lie JT, Kennedy RH, Elveback LR: Temporal arteritis. A 25-year epidemiologic, clinical, and pathologic study. Ann Intern Med 88:162, 1978.
398. Hamilton CR Jr, Shelley WM, Tumulty PA: Giant cell arteritis: including temporal arteritis and polymyalgic rheumatica. Medicine 50:1, 1971.
399. Hollenhorst RW, Brown JR, Wagener HP, Shick RM: Neurologic aspects of temporal arteritis. Neurology 10:490, 1960.
400. Bethlenfalvay NC, Nusynowitz ML: Temporal arteritis. A rarity in the young adult. Arch Intern Med 114:487, 1964.
401. Lie JT, Gordon LP, Titus JL: Juvenile temporal arteritis. Biopsy study of four cases. JAMA 234:496, 1975.
402. Bacon PA, Doherty SM, Zuckerman AJ: Hepatitis-B antibody in polymyalgia rheumatica. Lancet 2:476, 1975.
403. Bridgeford PH, Lowenstein M, Bocanegra TS, Vasey FB, Germain BF, Espinoza LR: Polymyalgia rheumatica and giant cell arteritis: histocompatibility typing and hepatitis-B infection studies. Arthritis Rheum 23:516, 1980.
404. Malmvall B, Bengtsson B, Kaijser B, Nilsson L, Alestig K: Serum levels of immunoglobulin and complement in giant-cell arteritis. JAMA 236:1876, 1976.
405. Liang GC, Simkin PA, Mannik M: Immunoglobulins in temporal arteries. An immunofluorescent study. Ann Intern Med 81:19, 1974.
406. Waller E, Tönder O, Milde E: Immunological and histological studies of temporal arteries from patients with temporal arteritis and/or polymyalgia rheumatica. Acta Pathol Microbiol Scand [A] 84:55, 1976.
407. Hazleman BL, MacLennan ICM, Esiri MM: Lymphocyte proliferation to artery antigen as a positive diagnostic test in polymyalgia rheumatica. Ann Rheum Dis 34:122, 1975.
408. Papaioannou CC, Hunder GG, McDuffie FC: Cellular immunity in polymyalgia rheumatica and giant cell arteritis. Lack of response to muscle or artery homogenates. Arthritis Rheum 22:740, 1979.
409. Liang GC, Simkin PA, Hunder GG, Wilske KR, Healey LA: Familial aggregation of polymyalgia rheumatica and giant cell arteritis. Arthritis Rheum 17:19, 1974.
410. Hazleman B, Goldstone A, Voak D: Association of polymyalgia rheumatica and giant-cell arteritis with HLA-B8. Br Med J 2:989, 1977.
411. Bell WR, Klinefelter HR: Polymyalgia rheumatica. Johns Hopkins Med J 121:175, 1967.
412. Healey LA, Wilske KR: Manifestations of giant-cell arteritis. Med Clin North Am 61:261, 1977.
413. Ballow SP, Khan MA, Kushner I: Giant-cell arteritis in a black patient. Ann Intern Med 88:659, 1978.
414. Cooke WT, Cloake PCP, Govan ADT, Colbeck JC: Temporal arteritis: a generalized vascular disease. Q J Med 15:47, 1946.
415. Ghose MK, Shensa S, Lerner PI: Arteritis of the aged (giant cell arteritis) and fever of unexplained origin. Am J Med 60:429, 1976.
416. Russell RWR: Giant-cell arteritis. A review of 35 cases. Q J Med 28:471, 1959.
417. Bevan AT, Dunnill MS, Harrison MJG: Clinical and biopsy findings in temporal arteritis. Ann Rheum Dis 27:271, 1968.
418. Hitch JM: Dermatologic manifestations of giant-cell (temporal, cranial) arteritis. Arch Dermatol 101:409, 1970.
419. Soderstrom CW, Seehafer JR: Bilateral scalp necrosis in temporal arteritis. A rare complication of Horton's disease. Am J Med 61:541, 1976.
420. Wagener HP, Hollenhorst RW: The ocular lesions of temporal arteritis. Am J Ophthalmol 45:617, 1958.
421. Gilbert GJ: Eyeball bruits in temporal arteritis. Dis Nerv Syst 31:130, 1970.
422. Fisher CM: Ocular palsy in temporal arteritis. Minn Med 42:1258, 1959.
423. Barricks ME, Traviesa DB, Glaser JS, Levy IS: Ophthalmoplegia in cranial arteritis. Brain 100:209, 1977.
424. Whitefield AGW, Bateman M, Cooke WT: Temporal arteritis. Br J Ophthalmol 47:555, 1963.
425. Hamrin B, Jonsson N, Landberg T: Involvement of large vessels in polymyalgia arteritica. Lancet 1:1193, 1965.

426. Barber HS: Myalgic syndrome with constitutional effects. Polymyalgia rheumatica. Ann Rheum Dis 16:230, 1957.
427. Hunder GG, Disney TF, Ward LE: Polymyalgia rheumatica. Mayo Clin Proc 44:849, 1969.
428. Fessel WJ, Pearson CM: Polymyalgia rheumatica and blindness. N Engl J Med 276:1403, 1967.
429. Bruk MI: Articular and vascular manifestations of polymyalgia rheumatica. Ann Rheum Dis 26:103, 1967.
430. Hamrin B, Jonsson N, Hellsten S: "Polymyalgia arteritica." Further clinical and histopathological studies with a report of six autopsy cases. Ann Rheum Dis 27:397, 1968.
431. Hamrin B, Östberg G: Polymyalgia arteritica. Acta Med Scand [Suppl] 533:1, 1972.
432. Fauchald P, Rygvold O, Øystese B: Temporal arteritis and polymyalgia rheumatica. Clinical and biopsy findings. Ann Intern Med 77:845, 1972.
433. Ettlinger RE, Hunder GG, Ward LE: Polymyalgia rheumatica and giant cell arteritis. Annu Rev Med 29:15, 1978.
434. Kansu T, Corbett JJ, Savino P, Schatz NJ: Giant cell arteritis with normal sedimentation rate. Arch Neurol 34:624, 1977.
435. Healey LA, Wilske KR: Anemia as a presenting manifestation of giant cell arteritis. Arthritis Rheum 14:27, 1971.
436. Hall GH, Hargreaves T: Giant-cell arteritis and raised serum-alkaline-phosphatase levels. Lancet 2:48, 1972.
437. Dickson ER, Maldonado JE, Sheps SG, Cain JA Jr: Systemic giant-cell arteritis with polymyalgia rheumatica. Reversible abnormalities of liver function. JAMA 224:1496, 1973.
438. Long R, James O: Polymyalgia rheumatica and liver disease. Lancet 1:77, 1974.
439. Von Knorring J, Wasastjerna C: Liver involvement in polymyalgia rheumatica. Scand J Rheum 5:197, 1976.
440. Klein RG, Campbell RJ, Hunder GG, Carney JA: Skip lesions in temporal arteritis. Mayo Clin Proc 51:504, 1976.
441. Albert DM, Ruchman MC, Keltner JL: Skip areas in temporal arteritis. Arch Ophthalmol 94:2072, 1976.
442. Wilkinson IMS, Russell WR: Arteries of the head and neck in giant cell arteritis. A pathological study to show the pattern of arterial involvement. Arch Neurol 27:378, 1972.
443. Fulton AB, Lee RV, Jampol LM, Keltner JL, Albert DM: Active giant cell arteritis with cerebral involvement. Findings following four years of corticosteroids therapy. Arch Ophthalmol 94:2068, 1976.
444. Klein RG, Hunder GG, Stanson AW, Sheps SG: Large artery involvement in giant cell (temporal) arteritis. Ann Intern Med 83:806, 1975.
445. O'Neill WM, Hammar SP, Bloomer A: Giant cell arteritis with visceral angiitis. Arch Intern Med 136:1157, 1976.
446. Hunder GG, Baker HL Jr, Rhoton AL Jr, Sheps SG, Ward LE: Superficial temporal arteriography in patients suspected of having temporal arteritis. Arthritis Rheum 15:561, 1972.
447. Moncada R, Baker D, Rubinstein H, Shah D, Love L: Selective temporal arteriography and biopsy in giant cell arteritis: polymyalgia rheumatica. Am J Roentgenol Radiat Ther Nucl Med 122:580, 1974.
448. Layfer LF, Banner BF, Huckman MS, Grainer LS, Golden HE: Temporal arteriography. Analysis of 21 cases and a review of the literature. Arthritis Rheum 21:780, 1978.
449. Morgan GJ Jr, Harris ED Jr: Prognostic implications of non-giant cell temporal arteritis. Arthritis Rheum 19:812, 1976.
450. Morgan GJ Jr, Harris ED Jr: Non-giant cell temporal arteritis. Three cases and a review of the literature. Arthritis Rheum 21:362, 1978.
451. Beevers DG, Harpur JE, Turk KAD: Giant cell arteritis — the need for prolonged treatment. J Chronic Dis 26:571, 1973.
452. Hunder GG, Sheps SG, Allen GL, Joyce JW: Daily and alternate-day corticosteroid regimens in treatment of giant cell arteritis. Comparison in a prospective study. Ann Intern Med 82:613, 1975.

453. Schneider HA, Weber AA, Ballen PH: The visual prognosis in temporal arteritis. Ann Ophthalmol 3:1215, 1971.
454. Nakao K, Ikeda M, Kimata S, Niitani H, Miyahara M, Ishimi Z, et al: Takayasu's arteritis. Clinical report of eighty-four cases and immunological studies of seven cases. Circulation 35:1141, 1967.
455. Fraga A, Mintz G, Valle L, Flores-Izquierdo G: Takayasu's arteritis: frequency of systemic manifestations (study of 22 patients) and favorable response to maintenance steroid therapy with adrenocorticosteroids (12 patients). Arthritis Rheum 15:617, 1972.
456. Lupi-Herrera E, Sanchez-Torres G, Marcushamer J, Mispireta J, Horwitz S, Vela JE: Takayasu's arteritis. Clinical study of 107 cases. Am Heart J 93:94, 1977.
457. Ishikawa K: Natural history and classification of occlusive thromboaortopathy (Takayasu's disease). Circulation 57:27, 1978.
458. Davy J: Researches, Physiological and Anatomical. Vol 1. London, Smith Elder and Co., 1839.
459. Savory WS: Case of a young woman in whom the main arteries of both upper extremities and of the left side of the neck were throughout completely obliterated. Med Chir Tr (London) 39:205, 1856.
460. Judge RD, Currier RD, Gracie WA, Figley MM: Takayasu's arteritis and the aortic arch syndrome. Am J Med 32:379, 1962.
461. Lupi E II, Sanchez G, Horowitz S, Gutierrez E: Pulmonary artery involvement in Takayasu's arteritis. Chest 67:69, 1975.
462. Wiggelinkhuizen J, Cremin BJ: Takayasu arteritis and renovascular hypertension in childhood. Pediatrics 62:209, 1978.
463. Ito I, Saito Y, Nonaka Y: Immunological aspects of aortitis syndrome. Jpn Circ J 39:459, 1975.
464. Ikeda M: Immunologic studies on Takayasu's arteritis. Jpn Circ J 30:87, 1966.
465. Ito I: Aortitis syndrome with reference to detection of antiaorta antibody from patients' sera. Jpn Circ J 30:75, 1966.
466. Ueda H, Saito Y, Ito I, Yamaguchi H, Sugiura M, Morooka S: Immunological studies of aortitis syndrome. Jpn Heart J 8:4, 1967.
467. Hirsch MS, Aikat BK, Basu AK: Takayasu's arteritis. Report of five cases with immunologic studies. Bull Johns Hopkins Hosp 115:29, 1964.
468. Strachan RW, Wigzell FW, Anderson JR: Locomotor manifestations and serum studies in Takayasu's arteriopathy. Am J Med 40:560, 1966.
469. Numano F, Shimamoto T: Hypersecretion of estrogen in Takayasu's disease. Am Heart J 81:591, 1971.
470. Naito S. Arakawa K, Saito S, Toyoda K, Takeshita A: Takayasu's disease: association with HLA-B5. Tissue Antigens 12:143, 1978.
471. Numano F, Isohisa I, Maezawa H, Juji T: HL-A antigens in Takayasu's disease. Am Heart J 98:153, 1979.
472. Isohisa I, Numano F, Maezawa H, Sasazuki T: HLA-Bw52 in Takayasu disease. Tissue Antigens 12:246, 1978.
473. Sasazuki T, Ohta N, Isohisa I, Numano F, Maezawa H: Association between Takayasu disease and HLA-DHO. Tissue Antigens 14:177, 1979.
474. Numano F, Isohisa I, Kishi U, Arita M, Maezawa H: Takayasu's disease in twin sisters. Possible genetic factors. Circulation 58:173, 1978.
475. MucKusick VA: A form of vascular disease relatively frequent in the orient. Am Heart J 63:57, 1962.
476. Lande A, Bard R, Rossi P, Passariello R, Castrucci A: Takayasu's arteritis. A worldwide entity. NY State J Med 76:1477, 1976.
477. Ask-Upmark E: On the pathogenesis of the hypertension in Takayasu's syndrome. Acta Med Scand 169:467, 1961.
478. Bonventre MV: Takayasu's disease revisited. NY State J Med 74:1960, 1974.
479. Ask-Upmark E: On the "pulseless disease" outside of Japan. Acta Med Scand 149:161, 1954.
480. Sandring H, Welin G: Aortic arch syndrome with special reference to rheumatoid arteritis. Acta Med Scand 170:1, 1961.
481. Sano K, Aiba T: Pulseless disease; summary of our 62 cases. Jpn Circ J 30:63, 1966.

482. Schrire V, Asherson RA: Arteritis of the aorta and its major branches. Q J Med 33:439, 1964.
483. Abe K, Miyazaki S, Kusaka T, Irokawa N, Aoyagi H, Otsuka Y, et al: Elevated plasma renin activity in aortitis syndrome. Jpn Heart J 17:1, 1976.
484. Cheitlin MD, Carter PB: Takayashu's disease. Unusual manifestations. Arch Intern Med 116:283, 1965.
485. Roberts WC, Wibin EA: Idiopathic panaortitis, supra-aortic arteritis, granulomatous myocarditis and pericarditis. A cause of pulseless disease and possibly left ventricular aneurysm in the African. Am J Med 41:453, 1966.
486. Cipriano PR, Silverman JF, Perlroth MG, Griepp RB, Wexler L: Coronary arterial narrowing in Takayasu's aortitis. Am J Cardiol 39:744, 1977.
487. Ayers MA: Takayashu syndrome and pregnancy: a ten year follow up. Am J Obstet Gynecol 120:562, 1974.
488. Hauth JC, Cunningham FG, Young BK: Takayasu's syndrome in pregnancy. Obstet Gynecol 50:373, 1977.
489. Asherson RA, Asherson GL, Schrire V: Immunological studies in arteritis of the aorta and great vessels. Br Med J 3:589, 1968.
490. Berkmen YM, Lande A: Chest roentgenography as a window to the diagnosis of Takayasu's arteritis. Am J Roentgenol Radiat Ther Nucl Med 125:842, 1975.
491. Kawai T, Yamada Y, Tsuneda J, Aoyagi T, Mikata A: Pleural effusion associated with aortitis syndrome. Chest 68:826, 1975.
492. Lande A, Rossi P: The value of total aortography in the diagnosis of Takayasu's arteritis. Radiology 114:287, 1975.
493. Tanaka H, Mihara K, Ookura H, Toyama Y, Sasaki H, Kashima T, Kanehisa T: Echocardiographic findings in patients with aortitis syndrome. Angiology 30:620, 1979.
494. Vinijchaikul K: Primary arteritis of the aorta and its main branches (Takayasu's arteriopathy). A clinicopathologic autopsy study of eight cases. Am J Med 43:15, 1967.
495. Lande A, Berkmen YA: Aortitis. Pathologic, clinical and arteriographic review. Radiol Clin North Am 14:219, 1976.
496. Inada K, Katsumura T, Hirai J, Sunada T: Surgical treatment in the aortitis syndrome. Arch Surg 100:220, 1970.
497. Sunamori M, Hatano R, Yamada T, Tsukuura T, Sakamato T, Suzuki T, et al: Aortitis syndrome due to Takayasu's disease. A guideline for the surgical indication. J Cardiovasc Surg 17:443, 1976.
498. Bloss RS, Duncan JM, Cooley DA, Leatherman LL, Schnee MJ: Takayasu's arteritis: surgical considerations. Ann Thorac Surg 27:574, 1979.
499. Turner A, Kjeldsberg CR: Hairy cell leukemia: a review. Medicine 57:477, 1978.
500. Golomb HM, Catovsky D, Golde DW: Hairy cell leukemia. A clinical review based on 71 cases. Ann Intern Med 89:677, 1978.
501. Naeim F, Gatti RA, Johnson CE, Gossett T, Walford RL: "Hairy cell" leukemia. A heterogeneous chronic lymphoproliferative disorder. Am J Med 65:479, 1978.
502. Hughes GRV, Elkon KB, Spiller R, Catovsky D, Jamieson I: Polyarteritis nodosa and hairy-cell leukemia. Lancet 1:678, 1979.
503. Rottino A, Hoffman G: A sarcoid form of encephalitis in a patient with Hodgkin's disease; case report with review of the literature. J Neuropathol Exp Neurol 9:103, 1950.
504. Rewcastle NB, Tom MI: Non-infectious granulomatous angiitis of the nervous system associated with Hodgkin's disease. J Neurol Neurosurgy Psychiatry 25:51, 1962.
505. Rosenblum WI, Hadfield MG: Granulomatous angiitis of the nervous system in cases of herpes zoster and lymphosarcoma. Neurology 22:348, 1972.
506. Greco FA, Kolins J, Rajjoub RK, Brereton HD: Hodgkin's disease and granulomatous angiitis of the central nervous system. Cancer 38:2027, 1976.
507. Rajjoub RK, Wood JH, Ommaya AK: Granulomatous angiitis of the brain: a successfully treated case. Neurology 27:588, 1977.
508. Magidson MA, Rajendran MM, Leutcher WM: Granulomatous angiitis of the central nervous system with an unusual angiographic feature. Surg Neurol 10:355, 1978.

509. Nurick S, Blackwood W, Mair WGP: Giant cell granulomatous angiitis of the central nervous system. Brain 95:133, 1972.
510. Razis DV, Diamond HD, Craver LF: Hodgkin's disease associated with other malignant tumors and certain non-neoplastic diseases. Am J Med Sci 238:327, 1959.
511. Schroeter AL, Copeman PWM, Jordan RE, Sams WM Jr, Winkelman RK: Immuno-fluorescence of cutaneous vasculitis associated with systemic disease. Arch Dermatol 104:254, 1971.
512. Dom CA, Chapman CG: Pseudo-Raynaud's: cryoglobulinemia secondary to occult neoplasm. Calif Med 95:391, 1961.
513. Hawley PR, Johnston AW, Rankin JT: Association between digital ischemia and malignant disease. Br Med J 3:208, 1967.
514. Friedman SA, Bienenstock H, Richter IH: Malignancy and arteriopathy. A report of two cases. Angiology 20:136, 1969.
515. Rubenstein MK: Mononeuritis in association with malignancy. Bull Los Angeles Neurol Soc 31:157, 1966.
516. Johnson PC, Rolak LA, Hamilton RH, Laguna JR: Paraneoplastic vasculitis of nerve: a remote effect of cancer. Ann Neurol 5:437, 1979.
517. Costanza ME, Pinn V, Schwartz RS, Nathanson L: Carcinoembryonic antigen-antibody complexes in a patient with colon carcinoma and nephrotic syndrome. N Engl J Med 289:520, 1973.
518. Sutherland JC, Markham RV Jr, Ramsey HE, Mardiney MR Jr: Subclinical immune complex nephritis in patients with Hodgkin's disease. Cancer Res 34:1179, 1974.
519. Theofilopoulos AN, Wilson CB, Dixon FJ: The Raji cell radioimmune assay for detecting immune complexes in human sera. J Clin Invest 57:169, 1976.
520. Teshima H, Wanebo H, Pinsky C, Day NK: Circulating immune complexes detected by ^{125}I-C1q deviation test in sera of cancer patients. J Clin Invest 59:1134, 1977.
521. Hellström I, Hellström KE, Sjögren HO, Warner GA: Serum factors in tumor-free patients cancelling the blocking of cell-mediated tumor immunity. Int J Cancer 8:185, 1971.
522. Ambrose KR, Anderson NG, Coggin JH Jr: Cytostatic antibody and SV40 tumour immunity in hamsters. Nature 233:321, 1971.
523. Price DL, Harris JL, New PFJ, Cantu RC: Cardiac myxoma. A clinicopathologic and angiographic study. Arch Neurol 23:558, 1970.
524. Burton C, Johnston J: Multiple cerebral aneurysms and cardiac myxoma. N Engl J Med 282:35, 1970.
525. Steinmetz EF, Calanchini PR, Aguilar MJ: Left atrial myxoma as a neurological problem; a case report and review. Stroke 4:451, 1973.
526. Damasio H, Seabra-Gomes R, da Silva JP, Antunes JL: Multiple cerebral aneurysms and cardiac myxoma. Arch Neurol 32:269, 1975.
527. Huston KA, Combs JJ Jr, Lie JT, Biuliani ER: Left atrial myxoma simulating peripheral vasculitis. Mayo Clin Proc 53:752, 1978.
528. New PFJ, Price DL, Carter B: Cerebral angiography in cardiac myxoma. Correlation of angiographic and histopathological findings. Radiology 96:335, 1970.
529. Cravioto H, Feigin I: Noninfectious granulomatous angiitis with a predilection for the nervous system. Neurology 9:599, 1959.
530. Budzilovich GN, Feigin I, Siegel H: Granulomatous angiitis of the nervous system. Arch Pathol 76:250, 1963.
531. Hughes JT, Brownell B: Granulomatous giant-celled angiitis of the central nervous system. Neurology 16:293, 1966.
532. Kolodny EH, Rebeiz JJ, Caviness VS Jr, Richardson EP Jr: Granulomatous angiitis of the central nervous system. Arch Neurol 19:510, 1968.
533. Vincent FM: Granulomatous angiitis. N Engl J Med 296:452, 1977.
534. Davis JA, Weisman MH, Dail DH: Vascular disease in infective endocarditis. Report of immune-mediated events in skin and brain. Arch Intern Med 138:480, 1978.
535. Wilkinson IMS: The vertebral artery. Extracranial and intracranial structure. Arch Neurol 27:392, 1972.
536. Castleman B, McNeely BU: Case records of the Massachusetts General Hospital. Case 41152. N Engl J Med 252:634, 1955.

537. Castleman B, McNeely BU: Case records of the Massachusetts General Hospital. Case 14-1967. N Engl J Med 276:741, 1967.
538. Hinck VC, Carter CC, Rippey JG: Giant cell (cranial) arteritis. A case with angiographic abnormalities. Am J Roentgenol Radiat Ther Nuc Med 92:769, 1964.
539. Harrison PE Jr: Granulomatous angiitis of the central nervous system. Case report and review. J Neurol Sci 29:335, 1976.
540. Walker RJ III, Gammel TE, Allen MB: Cranial arteritis associated with herpes zoster. Case report with angiographic findings. Radiology 107:109, 1973.
541. Gilbert GJ: Evidence of viral cause in granulomatous angiitis. Neurology 27:100, 1977.
542. Reyes MG, Fresco R, Chokroverty S, Salud EQ: Viruslike particles in granulomatous angiitis of the central nervous system. Neurology 26:797, 1976.
543. Rosenblum WI, Hadfield MG, Young HF: Granulomatous angiitis with preceding varicella zoster. Ann Neurol 3:374, 1978.
544. Linnemann CC Jr, Alvira MM: Pathogenesis of varicella-zoster angiitis in the CNS. Arch Neurol 37:239, 1980.
545. Arthur G, Margolis G: *Mycoplasma*-like structures in granulomatous angiitis of the central nervous system. Case reports with light and electron microscopic studies. Arch Pathol Lab Med 101:382, 1977.
546. Thomas L, Davidson M, McCluskey RT: Studies of PPLO infection. I. The production of cerebral polyarteritis by mycoplasma gallisepticum in turkeys; the neurotoxic property of the mycoplasma. J Exp Med 123:897, 1966.
547. Griffin J, Price DL, Davis L, McKhann GM: Granulomatous angiitis of the central nervous system with aneurysms on multiple cerebral arteries. Trans Am Neurol Assoc 98:145, 1973.
548. Snyder BD, McClelland RR: Isolated benign cerebral vasculitis. Arch Neurol 35:612, 1978.
549. Feasby TE, Ferguson GG, Kaufmann JCE: Isolated spinal cord arteritis. Can J Neurol Sci 2:143, 1975.
550. Judice DJ, LeBlanc HJ, McGarry PA: Spinal cord vasculitis presenting as a spinal cord tumor in a heroin addict. Case report. J Neurosurg 48:131, 1978.
551. Lyons EL, Leeds NE: The angiographic demonstration of arterial vascular disease in purulent meningitis. Report of a case. Radiology 88:935, 1967.
552. Dodge PR, Swartz MN: Bacterial meningitis — a review of selected aspects. II. Special neurologic problems, postmeningitic complications and clinicopathological correlations (concluded). N Engl J Med 272:1003, 1965.
553. Ferris EJ, Rudikoff JC, Shapiro JH: Cerebral angiography of bacterial infection. Radiology 90:727, 1968.
554. Wickbom GI, Davidson AJ: Angiographic findings in intracranial actinomycosis. A case report and consideration of pathogenesis. Radiology 88:536, 1967.
555. Suwanwela C, Suwanwela N, Charuchinda S, Hongsaprabhas C: Intracranial mycotic aneurysms of extravascular origin. J Neurosurg 36:552, 1972.
556. Buchanan DN, Walker AE, Case TJ: The pathogenesis of chorea. J Pediatr 20:555, 1942.
557. Rabinov KR: Angiographic findings in a case of brain syphilis. Radiology 80:622, 1963.
558. Solé-Llenas J, Pons-Tortella E: Cerebral angiitis. Neuroradiology 15:1, 1978.
559. Greitz T: Angiography in tuberculous meningitis. Acta Radiol (Diag) 2:369, 1964.
560. Lehrer H: The angiographic triad in tuberculous meningitis. A radiographic and clinicopathologic correlation. Radiology 87:829, 1966.
561. Dastur DK, Dave UP: Ultrastructural basis of the vasculopathy in and around brain tuberculomas. Possible significance of altered basement membrane. Am J Pathol 89:35, 1977.
562. Ferris EJ, Levine HL: Cerebral arteritis: classification. Radiology 109:327, 1973.
563. Wollschlaeger G, Wollschlaeger PB, Lopez VF, Zemel HJ: A rare cause of occlusion of the internal carotid artery. Neuroradiology 1:32, 1970.
564. Schigenaga K, Okabe M, Etoh K: An autopsy case of *Aspergillus* infection of the brain. Kumamoto Med J 28:135, 1975.
565. Davidson P, Robertson DM: A true mycotic *(Aspergillus)* aneurysm leading to

fatal subarachoroid hemorrhage in a patient with hereditary hemorrhagic telangiectasia. Case report. J Neurosurg 35:71, 1971.

566. Long EL, Weiss DL: Cerebral mucormycosis. Am J Med 26:625, 1959.

567. Merriam JC Jr, Tedechi CG: Cerebral mucormycosis. A fatal fungus infection complicating other diseases. Neurology 7:510, 1957.

568. Martin FP, Lukeman JM, Ranson RF, Geppert LJ: Mucormycosis of the central nervous system associated with thrombosis of the internal carotid artery. J Pediatr 44:437, 1954.

569. Courey WR, New PFJ, Price DL: Angiographic manifestations of craniofacial phycomycosis. Report of 3 cases. Radiology 103:329, 1972.

570. Acers TE: Herpes zoster ophthalmicus with contralateral hemiplegia. Arch Ophthalmol 71:371, 1964.

571. Selby G, Walker GL: Cerebral arteritis in cat-scratch disease. Neurology 29:1413, 1979.

572. Johnson RT, Richardson EP: The neurological manifestations of systemic lupus erythematosus. A clinical-pathological study of 24 cases and review of the literature. Medicine 47:337, 1968.

573. Feinglass EJ, Arnett FC, Dorsch CA, Zizic TM, Stevens MB: Neuropsychiatric manifestations of systemic lupus erythematosus: diagnosis, clinical spectrum, and relationship to other features of the disease. Medicine 55:323, 1976.

574. Trevor RP, Sondheimer FK, Fessel WJ, Wolpert SM: Angiographic demonstration of major cerebral vessel occlusion in systemic lupus erythematosus. Neuroraxiology 4:202, 1972.

575. Greenhouse AH: On chorea, lupus erythematosus, and cerebral arteritis. Arch Intern Med 117:389, 1966.

576. Brandt KD, Lessell S, Cohen AS: Cerebral disorders of vision in systemic lupus erythematosus. Ann Intern Med 83:163, 1975.

577. Andrianakos AA, Duffy J, Suzuki M, Sharp JT: Transverse myelopathy in systemic lupus erythematosus. Report of three cases and review of the literature. Ann Intern Med 83:616, 1975.

578. Ramos M, Mandybur TI: Cerebral vasculitis in rheumatoid arthritis. Arch Neurol 32:271, 1975.

579. Watson P, Fekete J, Deck J: Central nervous system vasculitis in rheumatoid arthritis. J Can Sci Neurol 4:269, 1977.

580. Watson P: Intracranial hemorrhage with vasculitis in rheumatoid arthritis. Arch Neurol 36:58, 1979.

581. Mandybur TI: Cerebral amyloid angiopathy: possible relationship to rheumatoid vasculitis. Neurology 29:1336, 1979.

582. Lee JE, Haynes JM: Carotid arteritis and cerebral infarction due to scleroderma. Neurology 17:18, 1967.

583. Estey E, Lieberman A, Pinto R, Meltzer M, Ransohoff J: Cerebral arteritis in scleroderma. Stroke 10:595, 1979.

584. Leonhardt ETG, Jakobson H, Ringqvist OTA: Angiographic and clinicophysiologic investigation of a case of polyarteritis nodosa. Am J Med 53:242, 1972.

585. Liebow AA: The J. Burns Amberson Lecture — pulmonary angiitis and granulomatosis. Am Rev Respir Dis 108:1, 1973.

586. Leeds NE, Rosenblatt R: Arterial wall irregularities in intracranial neoplasms. The shaggy vessel brought into focus. Radiology 103:121, 1972.

587. Leeds NE, Rosenblatt R, Zimmerman HM: Focal angiographic changes of cerebral lymphoma with pathologic correlation. A report of two cases. Radiology 99:595, 1971.

588. Margolis MT, Newton TH: Methamphetamine ("speed") arteritis. Neuroradiology 2:179, 1971.

589. Darmody WR, Thomas LM, Gurdjian ES: Postirradiation vascular insufficiency syndrome. Case report. Neurology 17:1190, 1967.

590. Kagan AR, Bruce DW, DiChiro G: Fatal foam cell arteritis of the brain after irradiation for Hodgkin's disease: angiography and pathology. Stroke 2:232, 1971.

591. Weiss EB, Forman P, Rosenthal IM: Allopurinol-induced arteritis in partial HGPRTase deficiency. Atypical seizure manifestation. Arch Intern Med 138:1743, 1978.

592. Shillito J Jr: Carotid arteritis: a cause of hemiplegia in childhood. J Neurosurg 21:540, 164.
593. Humphrey JG, Newton TH: Internal carotid artery occlusion in young adults. Brain 83:565, 1960.
594. Hilal SK, Solomon GE, Gold AP, Carter S: Primary cerebral arterial occlusive disease in children. Part I: Acute acquired hemiplegia. Radiology 99:71, 1971.
595. Harwood-Nash DC, McDonald P, Argent W: Cerebral arterial disease in children. An angiographic study of 40 cases. Am J Roentgenol Radiat Ther Nucl Med 111:672, 1971.
596. Kudo T: Spontaneous occlusion of the circle of Willis. A disease apparently confined to Japanese. Neurology 18:485, 1968.
597. Suzuki J, Takaku A: Cerebrovascular "Moyamoya" disease. Disease showing abnormal net-like vessels in base of brain. Arch Neurol 20:288, 1969.
598. Castleman B, McNeely BU: Case records of the Massachusetts General Hospital. Case 60-1966. N Engl J Med 275:1125, 1966.
599. Sprofkin BE, Blakey HH: Acute spontaneous cerebral vascular accidents in young normotensive adults. Arch Intern Med 98:617, 1956.
600. Stockman JA, Nigro MA, Mishkin MM, Oski FA: Occlusion of large cerebral vessels in sickle-cell anemia. N Engl J Med 287:846, 1972.
601. Taboada D, Alonso A, Moreno J, Muro D, Mulas F: Occlusion of the cerebral arteries in Recklinghausen's disease. Neuroradiology 18:281, 1979.
602. V Winiwarter F: Ueber ein eigentuemliche Form von Endarteriitis und Endophlebitis mit Gangrän des Fusses. Arch Klin Chir 23:202, 1879.
603. Buerger L: Thrombo-angiitis obliterans: a study of the vascular lesions leading to presenile spontaneous gangrene. Am J Med Sci 136:567, 1908.
604. McKusick VA, Harris WS: The Buerger syndrome in the Orient. Bull Johns Hopkins Hosp 109:241, 1961.
605. McKusick VA, Harris WS, Ottesen OE, Goodman RM, Shelley WM, Bloodwell RD: Buerger's disease: a distinct clinical and pathologic entity. JAMA 181:93, 1962.
606. Goodman RM, Elian B, Mozes M, Deutsch V: Buerger's disease in Israel. Am J Med 39:601, 1965.
607. Smolen JS, Youngchaiyud V, Weidinger P, Kojer M, Endler T, Mayr WR, et al: Autoimmunological aspects of thromboangiitis obliterans (Buerger's disease). Clin Immunol Immunopathol 11:168, 1978.
608. Gulati SM, Singh KS, Thusoo TK, Saha K: Immunological studies in thromboangiitis obliterans (Buerger's disease) J Surg Res 27:287, 1979.
609. Eisen ME, Tyson MC, Michael S, Baumann F: Adhesiveness of blood platelets in arteriosclerosis obliterans, thromboangiitis obliterans, acute thrombophlebitis, chronic venous insufficiency and arteriosclerotic heart disease. Circulation 3:271, 1951.
610. Craven JL, Cotton RC: Haematological differences between thromboangiitis obliterans and atherosclerosis. Br J Surg 54:862, 1967.
611. McLoughlin GA, Helsby CR, Evans LL, Chapman DM: Association of HLA-A9 and HLA-B5 with Buerger's disease. Br Med J 2:1165, 1976.
612. de Moerloose PH, Jeannet M, Mirimanoff P, Bouvier CA: Evidence for an HLA-linked resistance gene in Buerger's disease. Tissue Antigens 14:169, 1979.
613. Hill GL: A rational basis for management of patients with the Buerger syndrome. Br J Surg 61:476, 1974.
614. Hausner E, Allen EV: Cerebrovascular complications in thromboangiitis obliterans. Ann Intern Med 12:845, 1938.
615. Sachs IL, Klima T, Frankel NB: Transverse colon thromboangiitis obliterans. JAMA 238:336, 1977.
616. Williams G: Recent views on Buerger's disease. J Clin Pathol 22:573, 1969.
617. Fisher CM: Cerebral thromboangiitis obliterans (including a critical review of the literature). Medicine 36:169, 1957.
618. Wessler S, Ming S, Gurewich V, Freiman DG: A critical evaluation of thromboangiitis obliterans. The case against Buerger's disease. N Engl J Med 262:1149, 1960.
619. Shionoya S, Ban I, Nakata Y, Matsubara J, Shinjo K, Hirai M, et al: Diagnosis, pathology, and treatment of Buerger's disease. Surgery 75:695, 1974.

620. Shionoya S, Ban I, Nakata Y, Matsubara J, Hirai M, Miyazaki H, et al: Vascular reconstruction in Buerger's disease. Br J Surg 63:841, 1976.

621. Wong J, Lam STK, Ong GB: Buerger's disease — a review of 105 patients. Aust NZ J Surg 48:382, 1978.

622. Krahenbuhl B, Holstein P, Nielsen SL, Tonnesen KH, Lassen NA: Induced hypertension as a therapy in Buerger's disease (Thromboangiitis obliterans) Vasa 4:407, 1975.

623. Olsson AG, Thyresson N: Healing of ischaemic ulcers by intravenous prostaglandin E_1 in a woman with thromboangiitis obliterans. Acta Derm Venereol (Stockh) 58:467, 1978.

624. Kawasaki T, Kosaki F, Okawa S, Shigematsu I, Yanagawa H: A new infantile acute febrile mucocutaneous lymph node syndrome (MLNS) prevailing in Japan. Pediatrics 54:271, 1974.

625. Morens DM, O'Brien RJ: Kawasaki disease in the United States. J Infect Dis 137:91, 1978.

626. Tanaka N, Sekimoto K, Naoe S: Kawasaki disease. Relationship with infantile periarteritis nodosa. Arch Pathol Lab Med 100:81, 1976.

627. Carter RF, Haynes ME, Morton J: Rickettsia-like bodies and splenitis in Kawasaki disease. Lancet 2:1254, 1976.

628. Barbour AG, Krueger GG, Feorino PM, Smith CB: Kawasaki-like disease in a young adult. Association with primary Epstein-Barr virus infection. JAMA 241:397, 1979.

629. Krensky AM, Teele R, Watkins J, Bates J: Streptococcal antigenicity in mucocutaneous lymph node syndrome and hydropic gallbladders. Pediatrics 64:979, 1979.

630. Fossard C, Thompson RA: Mucocutaneous lymph-node syndrome (Kawasaki disease): probable soluble-complex disorder. Br Med J 1:833, 1977.

631. Weindling AM, Levinsky RJ, Marshall WC, Hood J: Circulating immune complexes in mucocutaneous lymph-node syndrome (Kawasaki disease). Arch Dis Child 54:241, 1979.

632. Hicks RM: Mucocutaneous lymph node syndrome in Hawaii. Arthritis Rheum 20:389, 1977.

633. Matsuda I, Hattori S, Nagata N, Fruse A, Nambu H, Itakura K, et al: HLA antigens in mucocutaneous lymph node syndrome. Am J Dis Child 131:1417, 1977.

634. Meade RH III, Keim DE, Cheeseman SH, LeClair JM, Modlin JF, Fiumara NJ, et al: Kawasaki syndrome — Massachusetts. Morbid Mortal Weekly Rep 29:369, 1980.

635. Darby CP, Kyong CU: Mucocutaneous lymph node syndrome. JAMA 236:2295, 1976.

636. Konishi Y, Tatsuta N, Miki S, Chiba Y, Kao C, Hikasa Y, et al: Mitral insufficiency secondary to mucocutaneous lymph node syndrome. A case report of successful surgical treatment. Jpn Circ J 42:901, 1978.

637. Fukushige J, Nihill MR, McNamara DG: Spectrum of cardiovascular lesions in mucocutaneous lymph-node syndrome: analysis of eight cases. Am J Cardiol 45:98, 1980.

638. Honda S, Matsumoto H, Mizoguchi Y, Hamasaki Y, Sunagawa H: Aortic regurgitation following acute febrile mucocutaneous lymph node syndrome (MLNS) in an infant. Jpn Circ J 43:463, 1979.

639. Yanagisawa M, Kobayashi W, Mutsuya S: Myocardial infarction due to coronary thromboarteritis, following acute febrile mucocutaneous lymph node syndrome (MLNS) in an infant. Pediatrics 54:277, 1974.

640. Kato H, Koike S, Tanaka C, Yokochi K, Yoshioka F, Takeuchi S, et al: Coronary heart disease in children with Kawasaki disease. Jpn Circ J 43:469, 1979.

641. Nitzkin JL, Hall CB, Berkowitz ID, Huntley CL, Rothenberg R: Kawasaki disease — New York. Morbid Mortal Weekly Rep 29:61, 1980.

642. Odom RB, Olson EG: Mucocutaneous lymph node syndrome. Arch Dermatol 113:339, 1977.

643. Hiraishi S, Yashiro K, Kusano S: Noninvasive visualization of coronary arterial aneurysm in infants and young children with mucocutaneous lymph node syndrome with two dimensional echocardiography. Am J Cardiol 43:1225, 1979.

644. Yoshikawa J, Yanagihara K, Owaki T, Kato H, Takagi Y, Okumachi F, et al: Cross-sectional echocardiographic diagnosis of coronary artery aneurysms in patients with the mucocutaneous lymph node syndrome. Circulation 59:133, 1979.

645. Yoshida H, Funabashi T, Nakaya S, Taniguchi N: Mucocutaneous lymph node syndrome. A cross-sectional echocardiographic diagnosis of coronary aneurysms. Am J Dis Child 133:1244, 1979.

646. Onouchi Z, Tomizawa N, Goto M, Nakata K, Fukuda M, Goto M: Cardiac involvement and prognosis in acute mucocutaneous lymph node syndrome. Chest 68:297, 1975.

647. Amano S, Hazama F, Hamashima Y: Pathology of Kawasaki disease: I. Pathology and morphogenesis of the vascular changes. Jpn Circ J 43:633, 1979.

648. Amano S, Hazama F, Hamashima Y: Pathology of Kawasaki disease. II. Distribution and incidence of the vascular lesions. Jpn Circ J 43:741, 1979.

649. Landing BH, Larson EJ: Are infantile periarteritis nodosa with coronary artery involvement and fatal mucocutaneous lymph node syndrome the same? Comparison of 20 patients from North America with patients from Hawaii and Japan. Pediatrics 59:651, 1977.

650. Ahlstrom H, Lundstrom N, Mortensson W, Östberg G, Lantorp K: Infantile periarteritis nodosa or mucocutaneous lymph node syndrome. A report on four cases and diagnostic considerations. Acta Paediatr Scand 66:193, 1977.

651. Smith AD: Infantile polyarteritis and Kawasaki disease. Acta Paediatr Scand 66:381, 1977.

652. Bergeson PS, Schoenike SL: Mucocutaneous lymph node syndrome. A case masquerading as Rocky Mountain spotted fever. JAMA 237:2299, 1977.

653. Everett ED: Mucocutaneous lymph node syndrome (Kawasaki disease) in adults. JAMA 242:542, 1979.

654. Schlossberg D, Kandra J, Kreiser J: Possible Kawasaki disease in a 20-year-old woman. Arch Dermatol 115:1435, 1979.

655. Milgrom H, Palmer EL, Slovin SF, Morens DM, Freedman SD, Vaughan JH: Kawasaki disease in a healthy young adult. Ann Intern Med 92:467, 1980.

656. Lee TJ, Vaughan D: Mucocutaneous lymph node syndrome in a young adult. Arch Intern Med 139:104, 1979.

657. Chesney PJ, Chesney RW, Purdy W, Nelson D, McPherson T, Wand P, et al: Toxic-shock syndrome — United States. Morbid Mortal Weekly Rep 29:229, 1980.

658. Kitamura S, Kawashima Y, Kawachi K, Fujino M, Kozuka T, Fujita T, et al: Left ventricular function in patients with coronary arteritis due to acute febrile mucocutaneous lymph node syndrome or related diseases. Am J Cardiol 40:156, 1977.

659. Sandiford FM, Vargo TA, Shih J, Pelargonio S, McNamara DG: Successful triple coronary artery bypass in a child with multiple coronary aneurysms due to Kawasaki's disease. J Thorac Cardiovasc Surg 79:283, 1980.

660. Kato H, Koike S, Yokoyama T: Kawasaki disease: effect of treatment on coronary artery involvement. Pediatrics 63:175, 1979.

661. Bluthe L: Zur Kenntnis des rezidivierenden Hypopyons. Inaugural thesis. Heidelberg, 1908.

662. Behçet H: Ueber rezidivierende Aphthose, durch ein Virus verursachte Geschwure am Mund, am Auge und de Genitalien. Dermat Wochenschr 105:1152, 1937.

663. Chajek T, Fainaru M: Behçet's disease. Report of 41 cases and a review of the literature. Medicine 54:179, 1975.

664. Shimizu T, Ehrlich GE, Inaba G, Hayashi K: Behçet disease (Behçet syndrome). Semin Arthritis Rheum 8:223, 1979.

665. Sezer FN: The isolation of a virus as the cause of Behçet's disease. Am J Ophthalmol 36:301, 1953.

666. Sezer FN: Further investigations on the virus of Behçet's disease. Am J Ophthalmol 41:41, 1956.

667. Evans AD, Pallis CA, Spillane JD: Involvement of the nervous system in Behçet's syndrome. Report of three cases and isolation of virus. Lancet 2:349, 1957.

668. Dowling GB, Dudgeon JA, Perkins ES: Discussion on Behçet's disease. Proc R Soc Med 54:101, 1961.

669. Sigel N, Larson R: Behçet's syndrome. A case with benign pericarditis and recurrent neurologic involvement treated with adrenal steroids. Arch Intern Med 115:203, 1965.

670. Gamble CN, Wiesner KB, Shapiro RF, Boyer WJ: The immune complex pathogenesis of glomerulonephritis and pulmonary vasculitis in Behçet's disease. Am J Med 66:1031, 1979.

671. Rogers RS III, Sams WM Jr, Shorter RG: Lymphocytotoxicity in recurrent aphthous stomatitis. Lymphocytotoxicity for oral epithelial cells in recurrent aphthous stomatitis and Behçet syndrome. Arch Dermatol 109:361, 1974.

672. Takano M, Miyajima T, Kiuchi M, Ohmori K, Amemiya H, Yokoyama T, et al: Behçet disease and the HLA system. Tissue Antigens 8:95, 1976.

673. Lehner T, Batchelor JR, Challacombe SJ, Kennedy L: An immunogenetic basis for the tissue involvement in Behçet's syndrome. Immunology 37:895, 1979.

674. Firat T: Results of immunosuppressive treatment in Behçet's disease: report of 55 cases. Ann Ophthalmol 10:1421, 1978.

675. Mamo JG, Baghdassarian A: Behçet's disease. A report of 28 cases. Arch Ophthalmol 71:38, 1964.

676. O'Duffy JD, Carney JA, Deodhar S: Behçet's disease. Report of 10 cases, 3 with new manifestations. Ann Intern Med 75:561, 1971.

677. Wolf SM, Schotland DL, Phillips LL: Involvement of nervous system in Behçet's syndrome. Arch Neurol 12:315, 1965.

678. O'Duffy JD, Goldstein NP: Neurologic involvement in seven patients with Behçet's disease. Am J Med 61:170, 1976.

679. Rosenthal T, Bank H, Aladjem M, David R, Gafni J: Systemic amyloidosis in Behçet's disease. Ann Intern Med 83:220, 1975.

680. Rosenthal T, Weiss P, Gafni J: Renal involvement in Behçet's syndrome. Arch Intern Med 138:1122, 1978.

681. Scarlett JA, Kistner ML, Yang LC: Behçet's syndrome. Report of a case associated with pericardial effusion and cryoglobulinemia treated with indomethacin. Am J Med 66:146, 1979.

682. Cadman EC, Lundberg WB, Mitchell MS: Pulmonary manifestations in Behçet syndrome. Case report and review of the literature. Arch Intern Med 136:944, 1976.

683. Lockhart JM, McIntyre W, Caperton EM Jr: Esophageal ulceration in Behçet's syndrome. Ann Intern Med 84:572, 1976.

684. Lehner T: Pathology of recurrent oral ulceration and oral ulceration in Behçet's syndrome: light, electron and fluorescence microscopy. J Pathol 97:481, 1969.

685. Lehner T: Progress report. Oral ulceration and Behçet's syndrome. Gut 18:491, 1977.

686. O'Duffy JD, Taswell HF: Blood transfusion therapy in Behçet's disease. Ann Intern Med 80:279, 1974.

687. Wolf RE, Fudenberg HH, Welch TM, Spitler LE, Ziff, M: Treatment of Behçet's syndrome with transfer factor. JAMA 238:869, 1977.

688. Cunliffe, WJ, Menon IS: Treatment of Behçet's syndrome with phenformin and ethyloestrenol. Lancet 1:1239, 1969.

689. Matsumura N, Mizushima Y: Leukocyte movement and colchicine treatment in Behçet's disease. Lancet 2:813, 1975.

690. Mizushima Y, Matsumura N, Mori M, Shimizu T, Fukushima B, Mimuro Y, et al: Colchicine in Behçet's disease. Lancet 2:1037, 1977.

691. Weinberger A, de Merieux P, Spitler L, Paulus H: Treatment of Behçet's syndrome with levamisole. Arthritis Rheum 23:760, 1980 (abstract).

692. Buckley CE III, Gills JP Jr: Cyclophosphamide therapy of Behçet's disease. J Allergy 43:273, 1969.

693. Aoki K, Sugiura S: Immunosuppressive treatment of Behçet's disease. Mod Probl Ophthalmol 16:309, 1976.

694. Bietti GB, Cerulli L, Pivetti-Pezzi P: Behçet's disease and immunosuppressive treatment. Our personal experience. Mod Probl Ophthalmol 16:314, 1976.

695. Huston KA, O'Duffy JD, McDuffie FC: Behçet's disease associated with a lymphoproliferative disorder, mixed cryoglobulinemia and an immune complex mediated vasculitis. J Rheumatol 5:217, 1978.

REFERENCES

696. Blomgren SE: Erythema nodosum. Semin Arthritis Rheum 4:1, 1974.
697. Fine RM, Meltzer HD: Erythema nodosum: a form of allergic cutaneous vasculitis. South Med J 61:680, 1968.
698. Winkelmann RK, Förström L: New observations in the histopathology of erythema nodosum. J Invest Dermatol 65:441, 1975.
699. Löfgren S, Wahlgren F: On the histo-pathology of erythema nodosum. Acta Derm Venereol (Stockh) 29:1, 1949.
700. Scott DG, Rowell, NR: Preliminary investigations of arteritic lesions using fluorescent antibody techniques. Br J Dermatol 77:211, 1965.
701. Wemambu SNC, Turk JL, Waters MFR, Rees RJW: Erythema nodosum leprosum: a clinical manifestation of the Arthus phenomenon. Lancet 2:933, 1969.
702. Schulz EJ, Whiting DA: Treatment of erythema nodosum and nodular vasculitis with potassium iodide. Br J Dermatol 94:75, 1976.
703. Wallace SL: Erythema nodosum treatment with colchicine. JAMA 202:144, 1967.
704. Cogan DG: Syndrome of nonsyphilitic interstitial keratitis and vestibuloauditory symptoms. Arch Ophthalmol 33:144, 1945.
705. Cogan DG: Nonsyphilitic interstitial keratitis with vestibuloauditory symptoms. Report of four additional cases. Arch Ophthalmol 42:42, 1949.
706. Haynes BF, Kaiser-Kupfer MI, Mason P, Fauci AS: Cogan syndrome: studies in thirteen patients, long-term follow-up, and a review of the literature. Medicine 59:426, 1980.
707. Cheson BD, Bluming AZ, Alroy J: Cogan's syndrome: a systemic vasculitis. Am J Med 60:549, 1976.
708. Agnello V, Koffler D, Eisenberg JW, Winchester RJ, Kunkel HG: C1q precipitins in the sera of patients with systemic lupus erythematosus and other hypocomplementemic states: characterization of high and low molecular weight types. J Exp Med 134:228, 1971.
709. McDuffie FC, Sams WM Jr, Maldonado JE, Andreini PH, Conn DL, Samayoa EA: Hypocomplementemia with cutaneous vasculitis and arthritis. Possible immune complex syndrome. Mayo Clinic Proc 48:340, 1973.
710. Marder RJ, Rent R, Choi EYC, Gewurz H: C1q deficiency associated with urticarial-like lesions and cutaneous vasculitis. Am J Med 61:560, 1976.
711. Curd JG, Milgrom H, Stevenson DD, Mathison DA, Vaughan JH: Potassium iodide sensitivity in four patients with hypocomplementemic vasculitis. Ann Intern Med 91:853, 1979.
712. Zeiss CR, Burch FX, Marder RJ, Furey NL, Schmid FR, Gewurz H: A hypocomplementemic vasculitic urticarial syndrome. Report of four new cases and definition of the disease. Am J Med 68:867, 1980.
713. McLean RH, Weinstein A, Chapitis J, Lowenstein M, Rothfield NF: Familial partial deficiency of the third component of complement (C3) and the hypocomplementemic cutaneous vasculitis syndrome. Am J Med 68:549, 1980.
714. Katz SI, Gallin JI, Hertz KC, Fauci AS, Lawley TJ: Erythema elevatum diutinum: skin and systemic manifestations, immunologic studies, and successful treatment with dapsone. Medicine 56:443, 1977.
715. Weidman FD, Besancon JH: Erythema elevatum diutinum. Role of streptococci, and relationship to other rheumatic dermatoses. Arch Dermatol Syphilol 20:593, 1929.
716. Macaulay WL: Erythema elevatum diutinum. Report ot a case. Arch Dermatol 79:202, 1959.
717. Scheie HG, Albert DM: Textbook of Ophthalmology, 9th ed. Philadelphia, WB Saunders Co, 1977.
718. Champion RH: Disorders affecting small blood vessels. Erythema and telangiectasia. In Rook A, Wilkinson DS, Ebling FJC (eds): Textbook of Dermatology, 2nd ed. Oxford, Blackwell Scientific Publications, 1972, p. 885.
719. Chusid MJ, Dale DC, West BC, Wolff SM: The hypereosinophilic syndrome: analysis of fourteen cases with review of the literature. Medicine 54:1, 1975.
720. Simon LS, Mills JA: Nonsteroidal antiinflammatory drugs (2 parts). N Engl J Med 302:1179, 1237, 1980.
721. Hazen PG, Michel B: Management of necrotizing vasculitis with colchicine.

Improvement in patients with cutaneous lesions and Behçet's syndrome. Arch Dermatol 115:1303, 1979.

722. Thorn GW: Clinical considerations in the use of corticosteroids. N Engl J Med 274:775, 1966.

723. Dale DC, Fauci AS, Wolff SM: Alternate-day prednisone. Leukocyte kinetics and susceptibility to infections. N Engl J Med 291:1154, 1974.

724. Fauci AS, Dale DC, Balow JE: Glucocorticosteroid therapy: mechanisms of action and clinical considerations. Ann Intern Med 84:304, 1976.

725. Axelrod L: Glucocorticoid therapy. Medicine 55:39, 1976.

726. Baxter JD, Rousseau GG: Glucocorticoid Hormone Action. New York, Spring-Verlag, 1979.

727. Fauci AS: Glucocorticosteroid therapy in clinical medicine. In Wyngaarden JB, Smith LH (eds): Cecil Textbook of Medicine, 16th ed. Philadelphia, WB Saunders Co. In press.

728. Rinehart JJ, Balcerzak SP, Sagone AL, LoBuglio AF: Effects of corticosteroids on human monocyte function. J Clin Invest 54:1337, 1974.

729. Fauci AS, Dale DC: The effect of in vivo hydrocortisone on subpopulations of human lymphocytes. J Clin Invest 53:240, 1974.

730. Fauci AS, Dale DC: Alternate-day prednisone therapy and human lymphocyte subpopulations. J Clin Invest 55:22, 1975.

731. Fauci AS: Mechanisms of corticosteroid action on lymphocyte subpopulations. II. Differential effects of in vivo hydrocortisone, prednisone and dexamethasone on in vitro expression of lymphocyte function. Clin Exp Immunol 24:54, 1976.

732. Butler WT: Corticosteroids and immunoglobulin synthesis. Transplant Proc 7:49, 1975.

733. Parrillo JE, Fauci AS: Mechanisms of corticosteroid action on lymphocyte sub-populations. III. Differential effects of dexamethasone administration on sub-populations of effector cells mediating cellular cytotoxicity in man. Clin Exp Immunol 31:116, 1978.

734. Haynes BF, Fauci AS: The differential effect of in vivo hydrocortisone on the kinetics of subpopulations of human peripheral blood thymus-derived lymphocytes. J Clin Invest 61:703, 1978.

735. Fauci AS: Alternate-day corticosteroid therapy. Am J Med 64:729, 1978.

736. Mussche MM, Ringoir SMG, Lameire NN: High intravenous doses of methylprednisolone for acute cadaveric renal allograft rejection. Nephron 16:287, 1976.

737. de Torrente A, Popovtzer MM, Guggenheim SJ, Schrier RW: Serious pulmonary hemorrhage, glomerulonephritis, and massive steroid therapy. Ann Intern Med 83:218, 1975.

738. Bacigalupo A, Giordano D, Van Lint MT, Vimercati R, Marmont AM: Bolus methylprednisolone in severe aplastic anemia. N Engl J Med 300:501, 1979.

739. O'Neill WM Jr, Etheridge WB, Bloomer HA: High-dose corticosteroids. Their use in treating idiopathic rapidly progressive glomerulonephritis. Arch Intern Med 139:519, 1979.

740. Neild GH, Lee HA: Methylprednisolone pulse therapy in the treatment of polyarteritis nodosa. Postgrad Med J 53:382, 1977.

741. Novack E, Stubbs SS, Seckman CE, Hearron MS: Effects of a single large intravenous dose of methylprednisolone sodium succinate. Clin Pharmacol Ther 11:711, 1970.

742. Gray D, Shepherd H, Daar A, Oliver DO, Morris PJ: Oral versus intravenous high-dose steroid treatment of renal allograft rejection. The big shot or not? Lancet 1:117, 1978.

743. Stubbs SS, Morrell RM: Intravenous methylprednisolone sodium succinate: adverse reactions reported in association with immunosuppressive therapy. Transplant Proc 5:1145, 1973.

744. Garrett R, Paulus H: Complications of intravenous methylprednisolone pulse therapy. Arthritis Rheum 23:677, 1980 (abstract).

745. Steinberg AD, Plotz PH, Wolff SM, Wong VG, Agus SG, Decker JL: Cytotoxic drugs in treatment of nonmalignant diseases. Ann Intern Med 76:619, 1972.

746. Schein PS, Winokur SH: Immunosuppressive and cytotoxic chemotherapy: long-term complications. Ann Intern Med 82:84, 1975.

747. Gershwin ME, Goetzl EJ, Steinberg AD: Cyclophosphamide: use in practice. Ann Intern Med 80:531, 1974.
748. Bagley CM Jr, Bostick FW, DeVita VT Jr: Clinical pharmacology of cyclophosphamide. Cancer Res 33:226, 1973.
749. Hill DL, Laster WR Jr, Struck RF: Enzymatic metabolism of cyclophosphamide and nicotine and production of a toxic cyclophosphamide metabolite. Cancer Res 32:658, 1972.
750. Hurd ER, Giuliano V, Ziff M: The effect of cyclophosphamide treatment on B and T-lymphocytes in patients with connective tissue diseases. Arthritis Rheum 16:554, 1973 (abstract).
751. Clements P, Levy J, Barnett EV: Immunosuppressive effects on B-lymphocytes in rheumatoid arthritis. Arthritis Rheum 16:537, 1973 (abstract).
752. Fauci AS, Dale DC, Wolff SM: Cyclophosphamide and lymphocyte subpopulations in Wegener's granulomatosis. Arthritis Rheum 17:355, 1974.
753. Fauci AS, Wolff SM, Johnson JS: Effect of cyclophosphamide upon the immune response in Wegener's granulomatosis. N Engl J Med 285:1493, 1971.
754. Stevenson HC, Fauci AS: Activation of human B lymphocytes. XII. Differential effects of in vitro cyclophosphamide on human lymphocyte subpopulations involved in B-cell activation. Immunology 39:391, 1980.
755. Steinberg AD, Daley GG, Talal N: Tolerance to polyinosinic-polycytidylic acid in NZB/NZW mice. Science 167:870, 1970.
756. Cupps TR, Silverman GJ, Fauci AS: Herpes zoster in patients with treated Wegener's granulomatosis: a possible role for cyclophosphamide. Am J Med 69:881, 1980.
757. Dinant HJ, Klippel JH, Decker JL, Balow JE, Plotz PH, Steinberg AD: Randomized trial of oral cyclophosphamide plus azathioprine and intravenous cyclophosphamide in lupus nephritis. Arthritis Rheum 23:666, 1980 (abstract).
758. Plotz PH, Klippel JH, Decker JL, Grauman D, Wolff B, Brown BC, et al: Bladder complications in patients receiving cyclophosphamide for systemic lupus erythematosus or rheumatoid arthritis. Ann Intern Med 91:221, 1979.
759. Johnson WW, Meadows DC: Urinary-bladder fibrosis and telangiectasia associated with long-term cyclophosphamide therapy. N Engl J Med 284:290, 1971.
760. Hansen HH, Muggia FM, Saini N: Cyclophosphamide and the urinary bladder. N Engl J Med 284:1043, 1971.
761. Johnson WW: Cyclophosphamide and the urinary bladder. N Engl J Med 284:1043, 1971.
762. Schilsky RL, Lewis BJ, Sherins RJ, Young RC: Gonadal dysfunction in patients receiving chemotherapy for cancer. Ann Intern Med 93:109, 1980.
763. Fosdick WM, Parsons JL, Hill DF: Long-term cyclophosphamide therapy in rheumatoid arthritis. Arthritis Rheum 11:151, 1968.
764. Warne GL, Fairley KF, Hobbs JB, Martin FIR: Cyclophosphamide-induced ovarian failure. N Engl J Med 289:1159, 1973.
765. Koyama H, Wada T, Nishizawa Y, Iwanaga T, Aoki Y, Terasawa T, et al: Cyclophosphamide-induced ovarian failure and its therapeutic significance in patients with breast cancer. Cancer 39:1403, 1977.
766. Miller JJ III, Williams GF, Leissring JC: Multiple late complications of therapy with cyclophosphamide, including ovarian destruction. Am J Med 50:530, 1971.
767. Fairley KF, Barrie JU, Johnson W: Sterility and testicular atrophy related to cyclophosphamide therapy. Lancet 1:568, 1972.
768. Kahn MF, Arlet J, Bloch-Michel H, Caroit M, Chaouat Y, Renier JC: Le risque de leucose aiguë après traitement des rhumatismes inflammatoires chroniques et des connectivites par les cytotoxiques à visée immunosuppressive. Rev Rhum Mal Osteoartic 46:163, 1979.
769. Weiss RB, Muggia FM: Cytotoxic drug–induced pulmonary disease: update 1980. Am J Med 68:259, 1980.
770. Lemmel E, Hurd ER, Ziff M: Differential effects of 6-mercaptopurine and cyclophosphamide on autoimmune phenomena in NZB mice. Clin Exp Immunol 8:355, 1971.
771. Johnson JP, Whitman W, Briggs WA, Wilson CB: Plasmapheresis and immunosuppressive agents in antibasement membrane antibody–induced Goodpasture's syndrome. Am J Med 64:354, 1978.

772. Rosenblatt SG, Knight W, Bannayan GA, Wilson CB, Stein JH: Treatment of Goodpasture's syndrome with plasmapheresis. A case report and review of the literature. Am J Med 66:689, 1979.

773. Erickson SB, Kurtz SB, Donadio JV Jr, Holley KE, Wilson CB, Pineda AA: Use of combined plasmapheresis and immunosuppression in the treatment of Goodpasture's syndrome. Mayo Clin Proc 54:714, 1979.

774. Lockwood CM, Rees AJ, Pearson TA, Evans DJ, Peters DK, Wilson CB: Immunosuppression and plasma-exchange in the treatment of Goodpasture's syndrome. Lancet 1:711, 1976.

775. Jones JV, Cumming RH, Bucknall RC, Asplin CM, Fraser ID, Bothamley J, et al: Plasmapheresis in the management of acute systemic lupus eyrthematosus? Lancet 1:709, 1976.

776. Wallace DJ, Goldfinger D, Gatti R, Lowe C, Fan P, Bluestone R, et al: Plasmapheresis and lymphoplasmapheresis in the management of rheumatoid arthritis. Arthritis Rheum 22:703, 1979.

777. Goldman JA, Casey HL, McIlwain H, Kirby J, Wilson CH Jr, Miller SB: Limited plasmapheresis in rheumatoid arthritis with vasculitis. Arthritis Rheum 22:1146, 1979.

778. Karsh J, Klippel JH, Plotz PH, Wright DG, Flye W, Decker JL: Lymphapheresis in rheumatoid arthritis: a randomized trial. Arthritis Rheum 23:701, 1080 (abstract).

INDEX

Note: Page numbers in *italics* refer to illustrations; page numbers followed by (t) refer to tables.